SOMATIC YOGA

FOR HEALING STRESS & TRAUMA

Reduce psychosomatic symptoms, enhance your mind-body connection, and overcome trauma with just 5 minutes of exercises each day.

Maia Solara

SUMMARY

If you are reading this book, it means you are seeking a path to healing and well-being. Somatic therapy is a world where the magic of the mind-body connection will lead you to make significant changes, discover your hidden potential, and triumph over past challenges.

Somatic healing is like a warm embrace for your entire being, recognizing and honoring the intricate dance between thoughts, emotions, and physical sensations. It is a gentle reminder that within you lies an incredible capacity for healing, waiting to be awakened. By tuning into the whispers of your body—the most subtle signals and movements—you can unlock a secret potential.

At the heart of somatic healing is the deep understanding that the body holds memories and emotions that sometimes manifest as physical discomfort or tension.

I am here to guide you step by step. Through simple yet powerful practices such as breath work, mindful movement, and body awareness exercises, we can tap into the wisdom stored in our bodies, releasing repressed tensions and old wounds.

But somatic healing is not just about finding relief from physical symptoms; it is a journey that takes us deep into the heart of our emotions and psyche. By engaging with our bodies in this way, we can gently bring forth buried emotions, memories, and beliefs, embarking on a beautiful journey of self-discovery.

When we embrace somatic practices and incorporate them into our daily lives, we begin to regulate our nervous system, increase self-awareness, and create a deeper connection with ourselves. It is through this integration that we experience true transformation, a newfound sense of resilience, and power over our health and choices.

In essence, somatic healing invites us to listen carefully to the wisdom of our bodies, honor its messages, and lovingly release any accumulated tension or trauma.

This book is an invitation to embark on a journey of self-discovery and profound well-being. It is a step towards realizing your deepest desires.

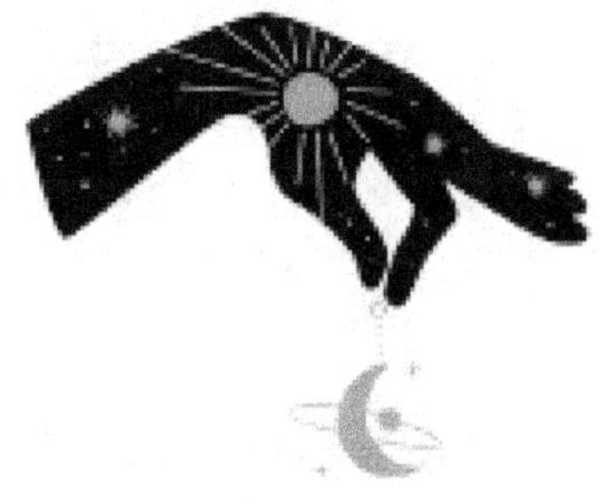

The mind-body connection is like a secret superpower, silently influencing our health and happiness. In the realm of somatics, where we explore this magical connection, we learn to harness it to heal, relieve stress, and improve our quality of life. Let's look at the 5 basics for understanding this incredible link and how it can fuel our personal growth and healing journey.

Seeing the Big Picture

Think of the mind and body not as separate entities but as best friends who are always communicating. Our thoughts, emotions, and beliefs have a direct link to our physical health, just as our physical state can influence our mental and emotional state.

Embracing this holistic view helps us see the bigger picture.

Emotions in the Body

Have you ever noticed that stress or past wounds can manifest as tension in your shoulders or as a knot in your stomach? It's the mind-body connection in action. Through somatic practices, we can dissolve these emotional knots stored in our bodies, paving the way for deep healing.

Rewiring for Healing

Our brains are incredibly adaptable, capable of rewiring based on our experiences. By engaging in somatic exercises focused on the mind-body connection, we can literally reprogram our brains, releasing stored trauma and making space for healing and growth.

Breathing to Connect

Breath is like a bridge between the mind and body, connecting them in perfect harmony. The practice of mindful breathing helps us tame emotions, calm nerves, and tune into physical sensations. It is a simple yet powerful way to enhance the mind-body connection.

Mindfulness in Movement

Mindfulness is not just about sitting and breathing but also about being fully present in our bodies. Embodied mindfulness takes this idea further, inviting us to tune into the sensations flowing through our bodies. Through this practice, we deepen our understanding of the mind-body connection and become more attuned to ourselves.

In essence, understanding the mind-body connection is like opening a hidden treasure chest of health and happiness. By embracing this link and practicing somatic exercises, we can tap into its transformative power and embark on a journey towards greater well-being.

Benefits of Somatic Exercises

Let's explore how somatic exercises can have a tangible impact on your life:

Increased Body Awareness: We have all experienced back or neck pain, often turning to medication or waiting for the pain to subside. But how often do we pause to reflect on the root cause of that pain? In today's fast-paced society, we are taught to seek quick fixes for symptoms rather than addressing the underlying issues. Medications may provide temporary relief but often mask the pain instead of addressing its source. Somatic practice encourages us to embrace, understand, and ultimately overcome pain by cultivating a deeper awareness of our bodies and their signals.

Improved Mind-Body Connection: How do you feel before an important meeting, exam, or challenging situation? Your mind might tell you to stay calm, but your body might react differently: sweaty palms, racing heart, sleep problems, headaches, or stomachaches. This conflict between mind and body is common. Somatic exercises bridge this gap, helping you unify the two realms so you can perform at your best in any situation.

Nervous System Regulation: Engaging in somatic techniques such as diaphragmatic breathing or grounding exercises can trigger the body's relaxation response, restoring a sense of peace and balance. You can distance yourself from feelings of anxiety, confusion, and fear while reconnecting with your inner calm and stability.

Emotional Processing: Have you ever felt stuck despite your efforts to achieve success? Do you struggle with following a diet? Have you started projects but never completed them? Do you desire a breakthrough in your work, but the right opportunity seems elusive? Unresolved emotions from past traumatic experiences might be holding you back, preventing you from fully realizing your potential. Somatic practices such as expressive movement or body scanning offer a pathway to explore, release, and find inner peace, clarity, and resolution.

In summary, by actively engaging in somatic exercises and listening to your body, you can embark on a journey towards healing trauma, reducing stress, and enhancing overall well-being!

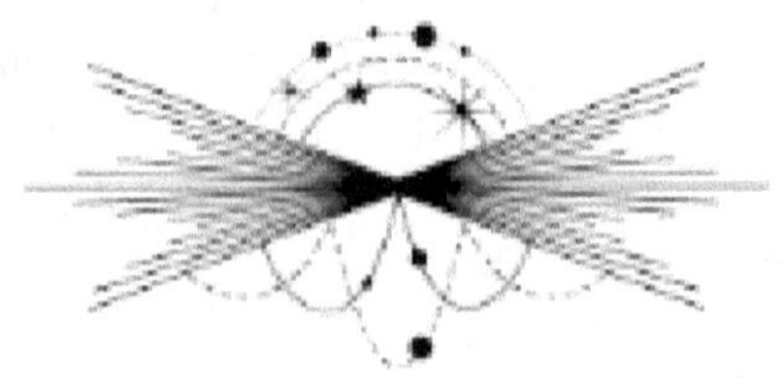

The Science Behind Somatic Healing

The roots of somatic care can be traced back to ancient healing practices that recognized the importance of addressing physical symptoms alongside emotional and mental states to achieve overall balance and harmony. In traditional healing systems, such as Ayurveda and Traditional Chinese Medicine (TCM), the concept of somatics was central to understanding health and well-being.

Ayurveda and the Doshas: Vata, Pitta, and Kapha

Ayurveda, originating over 5,000 years ago in India, is one of the oldest holistic healing systems. Derived from the Sanskrit words "Ayur" (life) and "Veda" (knowledge), it means "science of life." Based on ancient texts like the Charaka Samhita and the Sushruta Samhita, Ayurveda emphasizes balance and well-being through natural remedies, diet, herbs, and lifestyle practices.

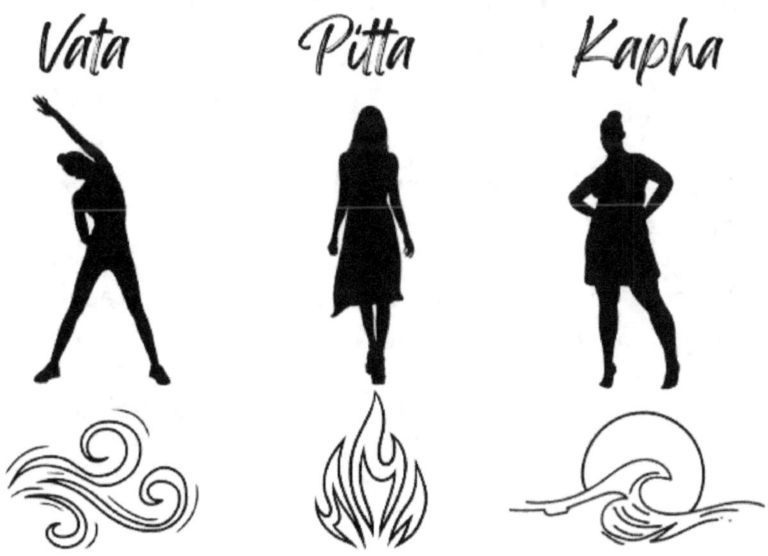

It identifies three doshas (Vata, Pitta, Kapha) and focuses on restoring their balance for health. The concept of dosha in Ayurveda represents three fundamental energies that govern physiological and psychological functions: Vata, Pitta, and Kapha.

Vata (Air and Ether) is characterized by the qualities of air and ether.

Role: Governs movement, including bodily functions such as breathing, circulation, and nerve impulses.

When in Balance: Vata fosters creativity, vitality, and enthusiasm. However, an excess of Vata can cause anxiety, restlessness, and digestive issues.

Qualities: Light, dry, cold, mobile, fast.

Balanced Vata Manifestations: Vitality, energy, creativity.

Balanced Psychological Vata Manifestations: Enthusiasm, quick thinking, flexibility.

Unbalanced Vata Manifestations: Anxiety, insomnia, constipation, digestive issues, dry skin.

Vata Balancing Tips:

> **Diet:** Warm, oily, and nourishing foods; avoid raw, cold, or dry foods.

> **Lifestyle:** Regular routines, warmth, relaxing activities like yoga and meditation.

> **Environment:** Warm and humid places, avoiding cold and windy conditions.

Pitta (Fire and Water) embodies the qualities of fire and water.

Role: Governs metabolism, digestion, and body transformation. This includes converting food into energy, regulating body heat, and managing emotions such as anger and ambition.

When in Balance: Pitta leads to intelligence, courage, and determination. However, an excess of Pitta can result in irritability, inflammation, and digestive issues.

Qualities: Hot, sharp, slightly oily, penetrating, luminous.

Balanced Pitta Manifestations: Good appetite, efficient digestion, radiant skin.

Balanced Psychological Pitta Manifestations: Intelligence, determination, courage.

Unbalanced Pitta Manifestations: Irritability, heartburn, inflammation, acne, excessive sweating.

Pitta Balancing Tips:

> **Diet:** Fresh, light foods; prefer sweet, bitter, and astringent flavors; avoid spicy, acidic, and salty foods.

> **Lifestyle:** Avoid excessive heat, practice relaxing activities, moderate exercise.

> **Environment:** Cool climates, avoid direct sun exposure.

Kapha (Earth and Water) represents the elements of earth and water.

Role: Governs structure, stability, and lubrication of the body. This includes tissue formation, growth, and mental and physical stability. A balanced Kapha promotes compassion, patience, and strength. However, an imbalance can lead to lethargy, weight gain, and respiratory issues.

Balanced Kapha Manifestations: Physical strength, resilience, robust immune system.

Balanced Psychological Kapha Manifestations: Calm, compassion, reliability.

Unbalanced Kapha Manifestations: Weight gain, lethargy, congestion, depression, and sluggish digestion.

Kapha Balancing Tips:

> **Diet:** Light, dry, and stimulating foods; avoid heavy, oily, or sweet foods.

> **Lifestyle:** Regular exercise, stimulating activities, and avoiding excessive sleep.

> **Environment:** Warm, dry environments; avoiding damp and cold conditions.

Traditional Chinese Medicine

Somatic therapy often draws inspiration from Traditional Chinese Medicine (TCM) and the concept of meridians. TCM views meridians as channels through which energy (called "qi" or "chi") flows to nourish the body's functions and organs. Any disharmony, whether physiological or emotional, is attributed to blockages or interruptions in the flow of energy along these meridians. In TCM, there are twelve main meridians, each corresponding to specific organs or functions of the body.

Dr. George Goodheart, founder of Applied Kinesiology, identified a relationship between the meridians and the major muscles. He discovered that by correcting muscle performance, the flow of energy along the associated meridians could be restored.

Dr. John Diamond expanded on Goodheart's work by developing the Emotional Acupuncture System (AES), which links meridians to emotional states. He observed that emotional states influence the flow of energy, potentially leading to disease. For example, Diamond, in collaboration with psychologists and cardiologists, found that many heart patients had difficulty managing anger. Anger creates a negative energy imbalance in the heart meridian, disrupting its flow over time and potentially leading to heart disease. Although not all angry individuals develop heart disease, Diamond's research indicates that most people with heart issues have experienced imbalances in the heart meridian related to anger.

Emotional imbalances often go unnoticed because they are repressed or unconscious. However, simple interventions, such as adopting positive attitudes, can restore the flow of energy.

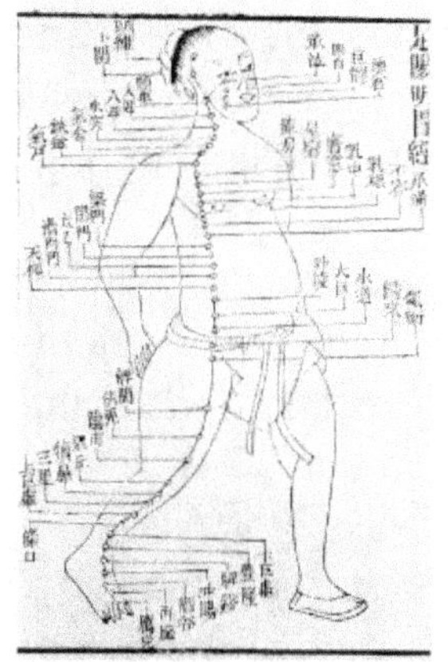
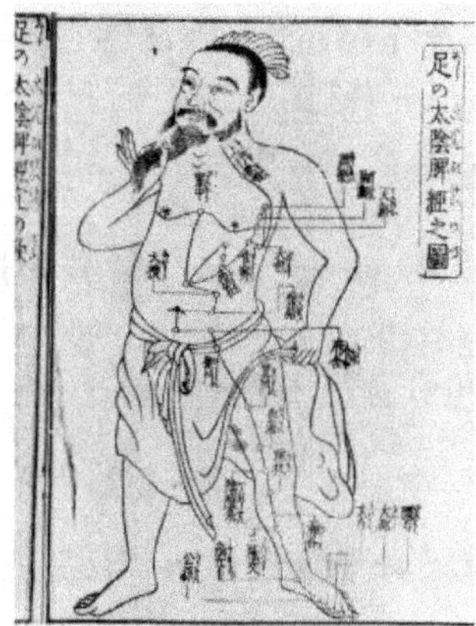

Kinesiological muscle tests show that positive affirmations, such as forgiveness, can strengthen weak muscles associated with imbalanced meridians, promoting health and well-being.

The 12 Energy Meridians i

Here is a list of the 12 energy meridians in Traditional Chinese Medicine (TCM):

- **Lung Meridian (LU)**: Responsible for regulating respiration and the distribution of Qi and bodily fluids. It starts from the chest area, travels down the arm, and ends at the thumb.

- **Large Intestine Meridian (LI)**: Associated with the elimination of solid waste from the body. It begins at the index finger, travels up the arm, and ends at the nose.

- **Stomach Meridian (ST)**: Governs digestion and the transformation of food. It starts from the eye, travels through the face, chest, and abdomen, and ends at the second toe.

- **Spleen Meridian (SP)**: Involved in the transformation and transport of nutrients and the regulation of blood. It starts at the big toe, travels up the leg and chest, and ends beneath the tongue.

- **Heart Meridian (HT)**: Regulates the blood and Qi of the heart, influencing the mind and spirit. It begins in the chest, travels down the arm, and ends at the little finger.

- **Small Intestine Meridian (SI)**: Responsible for the absorption and separation of fluids and nutrients. It starts at the little finger, travels up the arm, and ends at the ear.

- **Bladder Meridian (BL)**: Regulates fluid balance and urine release. It starts at the inner corner of the eye, travels along the back, and ends at the little toe.

- **Kidney Meridian (KI)**: Governs vital energy, growth, development, and reproduction. It starts from the sole of the foot, travels up the leg and abdomen, and ends in the chest.

- **Pericardium Meridian (PC)**: Protects the heart and regulates the flow of Qi in the chest. It starts from the chest, travels down the arm, and ends at the middle finger.

- **Triple Warmer Meridian (TE)**: Regulates Qi in the three warmers (upper, middle, and lower) and the distribution of fluids. It begins at the ring finger, travels up the arm, and ends at the head.

- **Gallbladder Meridian (GB)**: Affects decision-making and determination and regulates bile flow. It starts at the outer corner of the eye, travels along the side of the body, and ends at the fourth toe.

- **Liver Meridian (LR)**: Regulates the flow of Qi and blood, influencing emotions and digestion. It starts at the big toe, travels up the leg and abdomen, and ends in the chest.

These meridians are interconnected and work together to maintain energetic balance and overall health.

(Source: John Diamond, MD. Life Energy. 1985)

Meridians and chakras are closely interrelated elements within various holistic healing systems. While meridians are pathways through which energy flows in Traditional Chinese Medicine, chakras are energy centers within the subtle body according to Indian spiritual traditions, particularly within yoga and Hinduism. Chakras are believed to be centers of energy along the spine, with each associated with specific psychological, emotional, and spiritual functions. There are seven main chakras, ranging from the base of the spine to the crown of the head, and each corresponds to different aspects of human experience and consciousness. The term "chakra" in Sanskrit means "wheel" or "disk" and represents the vortex of energy believed to exist at each chakra point.

Both systems are integral to understanding and balancing the flow of energy in the body to promote health and well-being.

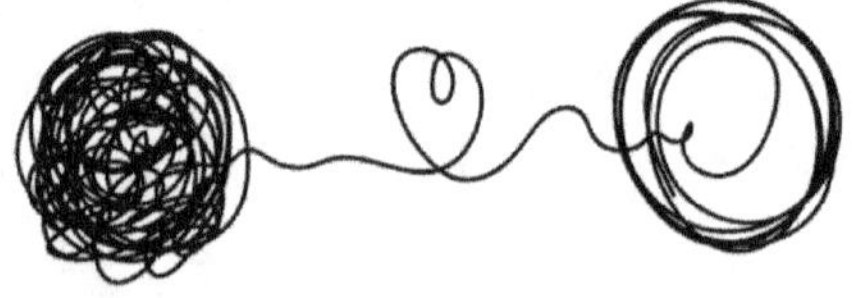

Stomach Meridian Disorders: Acid indigestion, Acid reflux, Allergies, Bags under the eyes, Bloating and gas, Digestive issues, Hunger, Mouth and lip sores, Neck pain, Nervous tension, Ovarian problems, Sinusitis, Sore throat, Stomach aches, Stomach ulcers, Tight chest, Weight problems.

Spleen Meridian Disorders: Allergies, Anemia, Blood-related issues, Carpal tunnel syndrome, Cysts, Diabetes, Edema (swelling), Fertility/pregnancy problems, Hypoglycemia, Immunodeficiency issues, Infections, Lymph nodes, Varicose veins, General weakness, Weight problems.

Heart Meridian Disorders: Angina, Arterial issues, Bleeding gums, Blood pressure (high or low), Chest pains, Circulation problems, Dizziness, Eczema, Heart issues, Sleep problems, Swollen glands.

Small Intestine Meridian Disorders: Abdominal issues or pain, Beer belly, Knee pain, Shoulder pain, Tinnitus / ear problems, Leg weakness.

Bladder Meridian Disorders: Ankle pain, Ankle weakness, Arthritis, Baldness, Back pain, Calf pain, Elbow issues, Fallen arches/flat feet, Headaches (especially at the front of the head), Joint pain, Nervous system problems, Osteoporosis, Sciatica, Scoliosis.

Kidney Meridian Disorders: Acne, Bone weakness, Bone pain, Lower back pain, Ear problems, Edema, Vision issues, Infertility/impotence, Prostate problems, Swollen ankles, Dental/gum issues.

Pericardium Meridian Disorders (circulation - sex): Hormonal issues, Impotence, Prostate problems, Sacral issues, Sexual problems, Painful breasts or nipples, Painful buttocks.

Triple Warmer Meridian Disorders: Adrenal exhaustion or fatigue, Allergies, Asthma, Diabetes, Fever, Hives, Hormonal problems, Hypoglycemia, Menopause, Mood swings, Premenstrual syndrome, Temper issues (too hot/cold), Weight problems.

Liver Meridian Disorders: Blurred vision, Candida, Eye infections, Eye diseases, Fungal diseases, Hepatitis, Hypertension, Jaundice, Low sperm count, Menopause, Premenstrual syndrome, Toenail problems (thick/yellow), Toxicity.

Gallbladder Meridian Disorders: Arthritis, Bitter taste in the mouth, High blood pressure, Gallstones, Hip or hip problems, Jaw or TMJ pain, Leg pain (especially on the sides), Migraines, Unilateral problems including headaches, Shingles, Teeth grinding.

Lung Meridian Disorders: Bronchitis, Chest infections, Colds, Cough, Flu, Pleurisy, Pneumonia, Respiratory issues, Shortness of breath, Skin problems, Tuberculosis.

Large Intestine Meridian Disorders: Colicky pains, Colon issues, Constipation, Hemorrhoids, Diarrhea, Herpes, Hip issues, Mineral deficiency, Nose issues, Toothache.

Identifying blocked meridians that cause disorders, diseases, or emotional disturbances is crucial for self-healing. Meridians act as energy highways, facilitating the transmission of neurological impulses and electronic signals throughout the body. These impulses regulate various biological processes, including those of the nervous and muscular systems. When meridians are obstructed, the flow of energy is hindered, leading to delays in transmission and actions. Alarm points along meridian segments indicate blockages and can lead to physical disturbances and, ultimately, degeneration and disease if not addressed. Maintaining clean meridians is essential for overall physical, emotional, and spiritual well-being, as it allows for timely intervention before disturbances evolve into diseases.

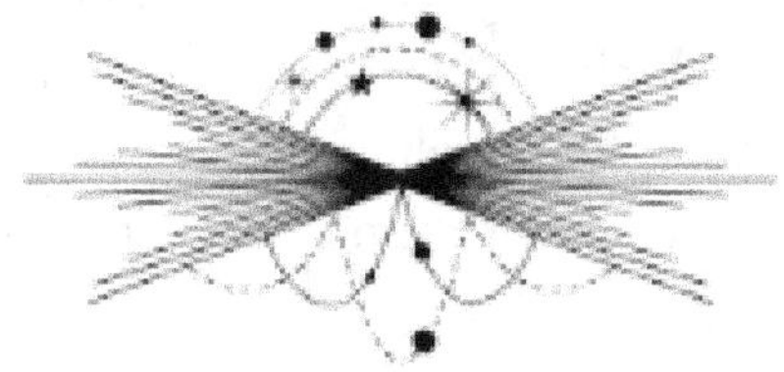

Just like meridians, blocked, stalled, or overactive chakras disturb the proper rotation of energy centers in the body. Chakras serve as energy centers through which meridians flow to recharge.

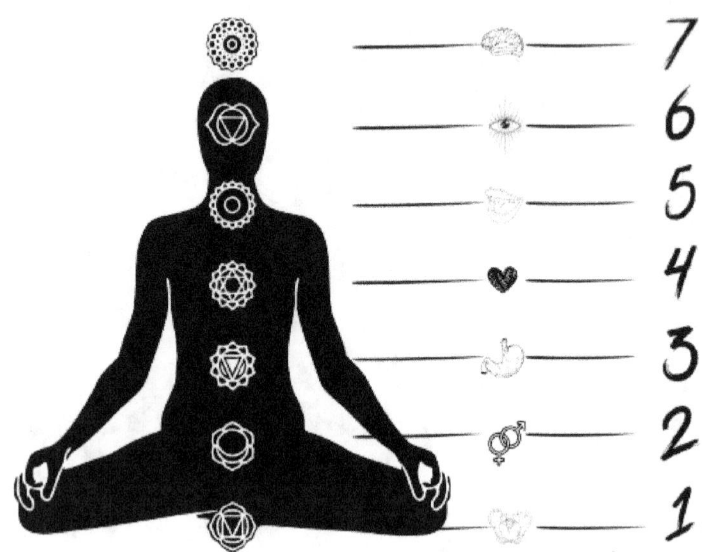

When chakras are stalled or overactive, the body's energy flow is heavily impacted, causing discomfort and agitation. However, when chakras are clear and aligned, and meridians have active and unobstructed energy flow, the body can heal effectively.

Which chakras and meridians regulate the healing of various disturbances? All, depending on the specific disturbance, the degree of meridian blockage, and the body's energy flow. Each meridian is associated with alleviating symptoms of different conditions related to muscles, organs, or biological processes.

1. Root Chakra (Muladhara Chakra)

- **Position:** Located at the base of the spine, around the sacrum.

- **Physical Body:** Connected to the colon, bones, muscles, and adrenal glands.

- **Emotional Being:** Linked to security, stability, safety, and primary needs such as housing and food.

2. Sacral Chakra (Svadhisthana Chakra)

- **Position:** Located below the navel.

- **Physical Body:** Connected to the sexual organs, bladder, kidneys, and reproductive glands.

- **Emotional Being:** Associated with sexuality, desire, creative energy, and emotions.

3. Solar Plexus Chakra (Manipura Chakra)

- **Position:** Located at the level of the navel, near the upper abdomen and sternum.

- **Physical Body:** Connected to the liver, adrenal glands, endocrine glands, and stomach.

- **Emotional Being:** Related to self-esteem, personal power, confidence, identity, and determination.

4. Heart Chakra (Anahata Chakra)

- **Position:** Slightly above the heart, in the center of the chest.

- **Physical Body:** Connected to the heart, lungs, and thymus gland.

- **Emotional Being:** Linked to love, joy, compassion, and forgiveness.

5. Throat Chakra (Vishuddha Chakra)

- **Position:** Located in the neck.

- **Physical Body:** Connected to the throat, mouth, and thyroid gland.

- **Emotional Being:** Associated with self-expression, communication, and authenticity.

6. Third Eye Chakra (Ajna Chakra)

- **Position:** Located at the center of the forehead, slightly above the eyebrows.

- **Physical Body:** Connected to the brain and pituitary gland. Often associated with physical issues such as headaches, nausea, and dizziness.

- **Emotional Being:** Linked to self-awareness, wisdom, imagination, and intuition.

7. Crown Chakra (Sahasrara Chakra)

- **Position:** Located above the crown of the head.

- **Physical Body:** Connected to the pineal gland, brain, and nervous system.

- **Emotional Being:** Associated with divine connection, higher consciousness, and spirituality.

Signs of Chakra Imbalance

Understanding the disturbances caused by blocked chakras highlights the importance of chakra cleansing. This practice not only ensures a smooth flow of energy from the earth through the body and head but also prevents physical disorders arising from energy blockages.

Signs that your Root Chakra is out of balance:

Immune system issues, blood or circulation problems, skeletal and bone problems, coccygeal nerve plexus issues, problems with legs, feet, and rectum, varicose veins, prostate problems, issues and tumors in the large intestine and rectum, depression, sciatica, hip, leg, and foot problems, frequent illnesses, immune disorders, anorexia, obesity.

Signs that your Sacral Chakra is out of balance:

Lack of awareness (material, financial, relational), difficulty expressing and sharing creativity and passion, sexual, reproductive, and childbirth issues, guilt or shame, blame or judgment, need for power and control over others, addiction problems, spleen issues, sexual organ problems, liver, upper intestine, kidneys, gallbladder, adrenal glands, pancreatic disorders or issues, central spine, back pain, gynecological problems, fibroids, uterine cysts, impotence, pelvic pain, libido and urinary problems.

Signs that your Solar Plexus Chakra is out of balance:

Insecurities and personal power issues, stress, fear, self-esteem, personality and ego problems, inability to listen to and trust one's own instinct/intuitive feelings, liver, mid-spine, pancreas, gallbladder, colon, spleen, small intestine, stomach and digestive system, diabetes, pancreatitis, hepatitis, colon diseases, cirrhosis, digestive system imbalances, intestinal tumors, eating disorders, hypoglycemia, chronic fatigue, hypertension, muscle spasms and disorders, adrenal fatigue, arthritis.

Signs that your Heart Chakra is out of balance:

Heart and circulatory system problems, blood issues, lungs, rib cage, diaphragm, thymus, breasts, esophagus, shoulders, arms, and hands, heart disease, breast and lung cancer, lung diseases, asthma, fluid in the lungs, shoulder, arm, and hand problems (carpal tunnel syndrome), immune disorders.

Signs that your Throat Chakra is out of balance:

Attitude, confidence, and self-expression issues, communication problems, fear of being judged and controlled by others, throat issues, dental problems, gum issues, thyroid problems, trachea issues, cervical vertebrae problems, esophagus, parathyroid and hypothalamus issues, throat cancer, swollen glands, dental and gum problems, laryngitis, chronic sore throat, thyroid problems, joint issues, addiction problems.

Signs that your Third Eye Chakra is out of balance:

Brain, neurological system, eyes, ears, nose, and pituitary and pineal glands, brain tumors, strokes, neurological disorders, blindness, dyslexia and learning disorders, deafness and ear pain, seizures, Alzheimer's, mental illnesses and personality disorders, sleep problems.

Signs that your Crown Chakra is out of balance:

Stagnation or resistance to change, denial of our spirituality, inability to trust life, selfishness, inability to achieve acceptance, affects overall health (physical, mental, emotional, and spiritual), depression, apathy, headaches, sensitivity to light and noise, allergies, multiple sclerosis, epilepsy, Parkinson's disease, senility, schizophrenia, paralysis or dizziness, dissociative states, panic disorders, nervous system problems.

Indeed, it is evident that different cultures recognize the importance of maintaining clarity and proper flow within our energy systems, including Meridians and Chakras, as crucial for supporting optimal physical, mental, emotional, and spiritual well-being.

In the modern context, somatic healing gained prominence in the mid-20th century through the work of pioneers such as Wilhelm Reich, Moshe Feldenkrais, and Alexander Lowen. These individuals developed therapeutic approaches that focused on the role of the body in processing and releasing emotional traumas, stress, and tensions. Their work laid the groundwork for contemporary somatic practices, now widely used to promote healing and well-being.

Wilhelm Reich (1897-1957), an Austrian psychiatrist, made significant contributions to the study of the mind-body connection in the early and mid-20th century. Initially a follower of Sigmund Freud, Reich later developed his own therapeutic approach, known as "character analysis." He emphasized the role of repressed emotions and sexual energy in psychological issues and sought to address them through therapy. Reich also introduced the concept of "orgone energy," proposing it as a vital force present in all living organisms. Reich theorized that orgone energy could exist in two forms: a positive one that promotes life (known as "positive orgone energy" or "POR") and a harmful, stagnant one (defined as "deadly orgone energy" or "DOR"). According to Reich, disruptions in the flow of orgone energy within the body can lead to physical and psychological disorders, while harmonious orgone flow supports vitality and health.

To harness and manipulate orgone energy for therapeutic purposes, Reich developed devices called "orgone accumulators." These boxes, made of layers of organic and inorganic materials, were believed to concentrate and amplify orgone energy, promoting healing and well-being.

Although Reich's theories on orgone energy remain controversial and have not been scientifically validated, they continue to provoke interest in alternative medicine and holistic healing practices.

Moshe Feldenkrais (1904-1984) was an Israeli physicist and judo expert who later became famous for his pioneering work in somatic education. His studies focused extensively on the mind-body connection. Feldenkrais developed the Feldenkrais Method, a form of somatic education that emphasizes mindful movement and awareness to improve physical functioning and overall well-being.

Through his method, Feldenkrais aimed to enhance awareness of one's movement patterns, habits, and posture. He believed that by increasing awareness of how we move and use our bodies, we could discover more efficient and comfortable ways of moving, leading to improved physical function and reduced pain.

At the heart of Feldenkrais' approach was the idea that our habits and movement patterns are deeply intertwined with our thoughts, emotions, and perceptions. By exploring and refining our movement habits through gentle and mindful exercises, we can create new neural pathways in the brain and improve our overall functioning.

Feldenkrais' work highlights the intricate relationship between mind and body, underscoring the importance of cultivating awareness and attention in movement to promote physical and psychological well-being.

Alexander Lowen (1910-2008), an American psychotherapist and founder of Bioenergetic Analysis, focused his studies on the mind-body connection. Lowen believed that psychological problems manifest physically in the body and vice versa, emphasizing the importance of addressing both aspects for holistic healing. Through his work in bioenergetics, a form of therapy that combines psychoanalytic principles with physical exercises to release emotional and physical tensions, Lowen helped individuals achieve greater self-awareness and overall well-being.

In Bioenergetic Analysis, developed by Alexander Lowen, there are five primary bioenergetic types, each characterized by distinct patterns of body structure, movement, and emotional expression:

1. Schizoid: Individuals with a schizoid bioenergetic type often exhibit a withdrawn and closed attitude, with a tendency to disconnect from emotions and physical sensations.

2. Oral: The oral type typically shows a pattern of dependency and seeking nourishment from others, often stemming from unmet infantile needs for love and security.

3. Psychopathic: Psychopathic types may display a rigid and defensive posture, with a particular focus on control and dominance. They may have difficulty expressing vulnerability or intimacy.

4. Masochistic: Masochistic types tend to hold tension in their bodies, often showing a hunched or collapsed posture. They may struggle with assertiveness and may harbor feelings of guilt or self-blame.

5. Rigid: Rigid types often present with a tense and constricted body posture, reflecting a strong need for control and perfectionism. They may have issues with flexibility and adaptability both physically and emotionally.

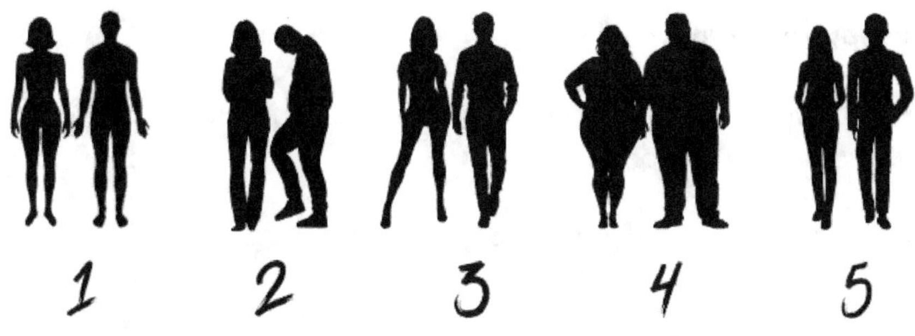

These bioenergetic types provide a framework for understanding the interaction between physical and psychological aspects of personality, guiding therapeutic interventions aimed at promoting greater self-awareness and healing.

Balancing the 5 bioenergetic types involves understanding and addressing the specific physical and psychological characteristics associated with each type. Here is a brief overview of how to balance each type:

Schizoid Type:

- Encourage grounding activities, such as walking or gardening.

- Foster emotional expression through journaling or talking with a trusted friend.

- Practice relaxation techniques like deep breathing or meditation to calm the mind.

Oral Type:

- Cultivate self-compassion and practice setting boundaries in relationships.

- Engage in activities that promote self-nourishment and care.

- Explore creative outlets such as art, music, or writing to express emotions.

Psychopathic Type:

- Develop empathy and emotional awareness through therapy or self-reflection.

- Practice assertiveness and boundary-setting in relationships.

- Engage in activities that promote self-awareness and responsibility.

Masochistic Type:

- Challenge self-limiting beliefs and negative self-talk through cognitive-behavioral techniques.

- Promote self-compassion and self-care practices.

- Explore activities that encourage self-expression and assertiveness.

Rigid Type:

- Cultivate flexibility and openness to new experiences.

- Practice relaxation techniques to release physical tension and stress.

- Engage in activities that promote creativity and spontaneity.

These are general guidelines, and personalized approaches may be necessary for each individual. Consulting a qualified therapist or a practitioner trained in bioenergetics or Ayurveda can provide tailored guidance for effectively balancing these types.

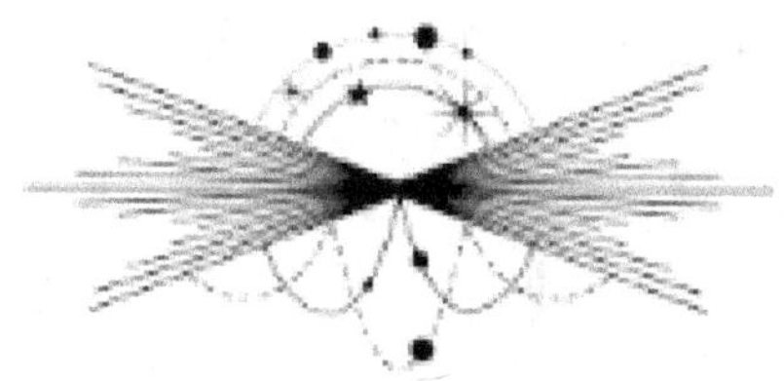

The book you are currently reading draws inspiration from traditional medicine and contemporary studies, such as those described in *The Body Keeps the Score*. This narrative explores the journey of therapists and scientists who integrate brain science, attachment research, and body awareness into trauma treatments, aiming to liberate people from past traumas. Leveraging the brain's neuroplasticity, these therapies seek to rewire disrupted functioning and restore individuals' ability to understand and experience their emotions. They offer experiences that counter feelings of powerlessness and invisibility associated with trauma, allowing survivors to reclaim their bodies and their lives.

Bessel van der Kolk, author of *The Body Keeps the Score*, based on decades of research and clinical practice, reveals how trauma fundamentally reshapes both the brain and the body. He explores why traumatized individuals experience anxiety, numbness, anger, and difficulties with concentration, memory, and relationship building. The author's unique perspective as both a scientific researcher and a practicing therapist provides a deeply personal and analytical approach to trauma recovery, making the book highly engaging and emotionally impactful.

The title, *The Body Keeps the Score*, underscores the central concept that exposure to trauma leads to the development of an overactive alarm system and physical responses locked in fight/flight/freeze mode. Trauma alters the brain circuits involved in concentration, flexibility, and emotional regulation, perpetuating a sense of danger and powerlessness. This continuous release of stress hormones damages the immune system and organ function. The key to lasting healing lies in creating safety for trauma survivors to inhabit their bodies, feel their emotions, and understand their experiences. This requires significant affection, acceptance, and warmth. Various therapeutic approaches tailored to individual needs, including trauma processing, neurofeedback, theater, meditation, play, and yoga, are used.

Readers will be inspired by human resilience and the transformative power of relationships, both personal and communal, to provide support and facilitate healing.

EMDR Therapy for Overcoming Trauma

A therapy that strongly demonstrates the interconnectedness of body and mind is Eye Movement Desensitization and Reprocessing (EMDR) therapy.

EMDR was developed by Francine Shapiro in the late 1980s. Shapiro, an American psychologist, initially discovered the therapeutic potential of eye movements in processing distressing memories during a walk in the park. She observed that moving her eyes back and forth seemed to alleviate the negative emotions associated with troubling thoughts.

EMDR has become one of the most widely used therapies for overcoming trauma, as it achieves excellent results in a very short time. It is a psychotherapeutic approach that integrates elements of cognitive therapy, exposure therapy, and bilateral stimulation to help people process traumatic memories and experiences. It involves a structured eight-phase protocol designed to address past experiences, current triggers, and future challenges related to trauma. During EMDR sessions, patients recall distressing memories

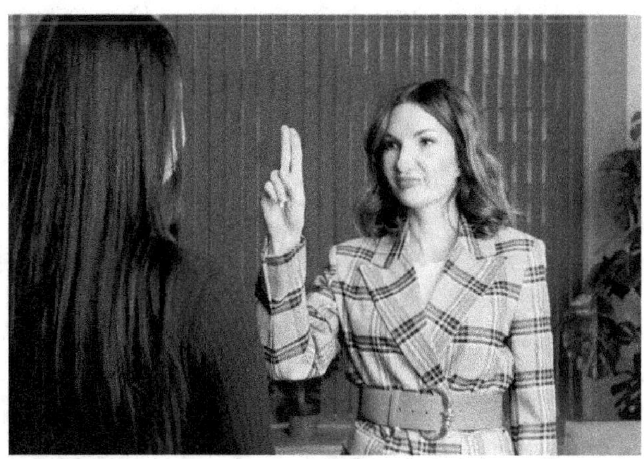

while simultaneously undergoing bilateral stimulation, such as following the therapist's fingers with their eyes or listening to alternating sounds or tactile sensations.

The goal of EMDR therapy is to facilitate the reprocessing of traumatic memories, allowing individuals to integrate these experiences into their broader autobiographical memory network in a more adaptive and less distressing way. EMDR has been extensively studied and is recognized as an effective treatment for post-traumatic stress disorder (PTSD) and other trauma-related conditions. It is used by mental health professionals worldwide to help individuals recover from the psychological effects of trauma and lead healthier, more fulfilling lives.

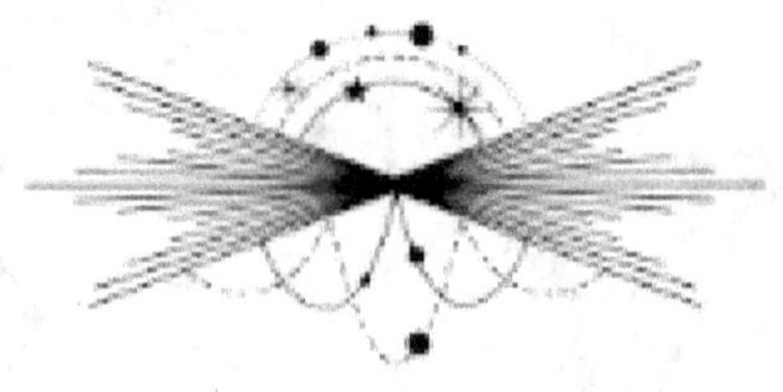

"Trauma is not the story of something that happened then. It is the imprint of pain, horror, and fear that lives in people now." – Bessel van der Kolk

It is crucial to recognize that trauma is a common human experience that can be addressed and overcome. Understanding the complexities of trauma is the first step toward healing and reclaiming one's well-being. This book aims to guide you step by step through the process of facing and overcoming the pain and fear associated with trauma. We explore how trauma manifests in the body and mind and how we can address its effects to cultivate resilience and healing.

What is Trauma?

Bessel van der Kolk defines trauma as an experience that overwhelms an individual's ability to cope with the situation, leaving them feeling helpless, powerless, and deeply insecure. Trauma can stem from various events, including but not limited to physical or sexual abuse, neglect, accidents, natural disasters, violence, or witnessed violence. Van der Kolk emphasizes that trauma is not just an event but also the lasting impact it has on an individual's emotional, psychological, and physical well-being, often altering one's sense of self, relationships, and overall functioning.

Types of Trauma

There are six main types of trauma:

1. **Acute Trauma**: Results from a single traumatic event, such as a car accident or a natural disaster.

2. **Chronic Trauma**: Stems from prolonged exposure to stressors, such as domestic violence or ongoing abuse.

3. **Complex Trauma**: Includes the cumulative impact of multiple traumatic experiences, often occurring within interpersonal relationships or systems of oppression.

4. **Developmental Trauma**: Arises from negative experiences during critical periods of childhood development, such as abandonment or disruptions in attachment.

5. **Intergenerational Trauma**: Transmitted through generations, often due to historical events such as genocide, slavery, or forced displacement.

6. **Vicarious Trauma**: Indirect experience through exposure to others' trauma, commonly seen in professions like healthcare, emergency response, and social work.

Therapists also use the distinction between "Big T" trauma and "Small t" trauma to differentiate between types and severity of traumatic experiences:

- **Big T Trauma**: Refers to significant or major traumatic events that represent a serious threat to a person's life or physical integrity. Examples include natural disasters, combat exposure, sexual violence, severe accidents, or acts of terrorism. These events often have a profound and immediate impact on an individual's sense of safety, well-being, and functioning.

- **Small t Trauma**: Refers to less severe or less obvious traumatic experiences that can still significantly affect an individual's emotional and psychological well-being. Examples include emotional neglect, verbal abuse, chronic stress, bullying, or ongoing family dysfunction. Although these experiences do not represent an immediate threat to physical safety, they can cause enduring emotional distress and contribute to the development of mental health issues like anxiety, depression, or PTSD.

Small t traumas are often cumulative and can occur over an extended period, gradually eroding an individual's sense of safety and self-esteem.

Therapists use the distinction between Big T and small t trauma to tailor interventions and therapeutic approaches to their clients' specific needs. While Big T trauma may require more intensive and specialized interventions to address immediate safety concerns and trauma symptoms, small t trauma may benefit from supportive therapy aimed at processing emotions, building coping skills, and fostering resilience.

Manifestations of Trauma

Trauma can manifest in the body in various ways, affecting both physical and psychological well-being. Some common manifestations of trauma in the body include:

- **Hyperarousal**: Individuals may experience heightened states of arousal, characterized by increased heart rate, hypervigilance, and an exaggerated startle response. This state of hyperarousal can lead to feelings of anxiety, agitation, and difficulty relaxing or sleeping.

- **Hypervigilance**: Trauma survivors may remain in a state of heightened alertness for potential threats, constantly scanning their environment for signs of danger. This state of hypervigilance can contribute to feelings of stress, fatigue, and an inability to feel safe or comfortable.

- **Physical Symptoms**: Trauma can also manifest as physical symptoms such as headaches, muscle tension, gastrointestinal problems, and chronic pain. These physical symptoms can result from the body's physiological response to stress and trauma, including the release of stress hormones like cortisol and adrenaline.

- **Somatic Symptoms**: Trauma may be stored in the body as somatic sensations, leading to feelings of discomfort, numbness, or tension in specific areas. People may experience sensations like chest tightness, stomach knots, or a sense of heaviness or constriction.

- **Dissociation**: In response to overwhelming trauma, some individuals may dissociate, disconnecting from physical sensations, emotions, or the surrounding environment as a means of self-preservation. Dissociation can manifest as a sense of detachment from one's body, memory gaps, or a feeling that the world is unreal or distorted.

- **Impact on the Nervous System**: Trauma can dysregulate the nervous system, causing disruptions in the body's stress response system. This dysregulation can lead to symptoms such as difficulty regulating emotions, mood swings, and increased sensitivity to stressors.

In general, trauma can have profound effects on the body, influencing both physical health and psychological well-being. It is essential for those who have experienced trauma to seek support from mental health professionals who can help them process and address these impacts.

Somatic Therapy

Let's delve into the essence of the book: somatic therapy. This therapeutic approach recognizes the intricate connection between mind and body, acknowledging that traumatic experiences are stored not only in the mind but also in the physical body. Somatic therapy aims to address trauma by focusing on bodily sensations, movements, and experiences.

What is Somatic Therapy?

Somatic therapy is a transformative practice that delves deeply into the core of our being, offering a journey of self-discovery and realignment. It is practiced through various modalities, including yoga, movement therapy, mindfulness techniques, breathwork, body awareness exercises, and somatic experiencing. Through this method, we explore the intricate connections between mind, body, and spirit, seeking harmony and balance within ourselves.

The Therapeutic Process

The therapeutic process generally follows several fundamental stages:

1. **Body Awareness**: The first step involves cultivating awareness of bodily sensations and experiences. Individuals are encouraged to notice physical sensations, tensions, and areas of discomfort in their bodies, often through mindfulness practices or guided exercises.

2. **Sensation Tracking**: The person learns to track the sensations and bodily responses associated with past traumatic experiences. This may involve identifying areas of

tension, changes in breathing patterns, or specific physical sensations that emerge when recalling traumatic memories.

3. **Somatic Resources**: Therapists help individuals develop somatic resources to regulate their nervous systems and manage discomforting emotions. This may include techniques such as grounding exercises, breathwork, or physical movements to promote relaxation and safety.

4. **Somatic Processing**: Individuals engage in somatic processing to explore and release trauma stored in the body. This may involve gently revisiting traumatic memories while paying attention to bodily sensations, allowing for the gradual processing and integration of past experiences.

5. **Integration and Regulation**: The final phase focuses on integrating the insights and experiences gained through somatic therapy into daily life. Clients learn to regulate their nervous systems, manage triggers, and cultivate resilience throughout their healing journey.

Through these stages, somatic therapy offers a holistic approach to trauma recovery, addressing the interaction between mind, body, and spirit in the healing process.

Body Awareness

Body awareness in somatic therapy involves developing a deep understanding of the sensations and experiences stored in the physical body. One technique used to enhance body awareness is creating a somatic map, which serves as a visual representation of where emotions and sensations are held in the body and how they feel. In this exercise, individuals are guided to identify and describe bodily sensations using descriptors such as tight, compressed, light, or heavy. These descriptors help pinpoint specific areas of tension or discomfort, facilitating a more nuanced understanding of bodily experiences. It is important to note that somatic map descriptors typically focus on physical sensations rather than cognitive or emotional states, allowing individuals to connect more deeply with their bodily experiences without the influence of cognitive interpretations. Through the process of creating and exploring somatic maps, individuals can gain valuable insights into the connection between their emotions, sensations, and physical body, ultimately supporting the healing process in somatic therapy.

Somatic Maps

These are examples of somatic maps. Note that the figure is represented both front and back, as attention is needed for every part of the body.

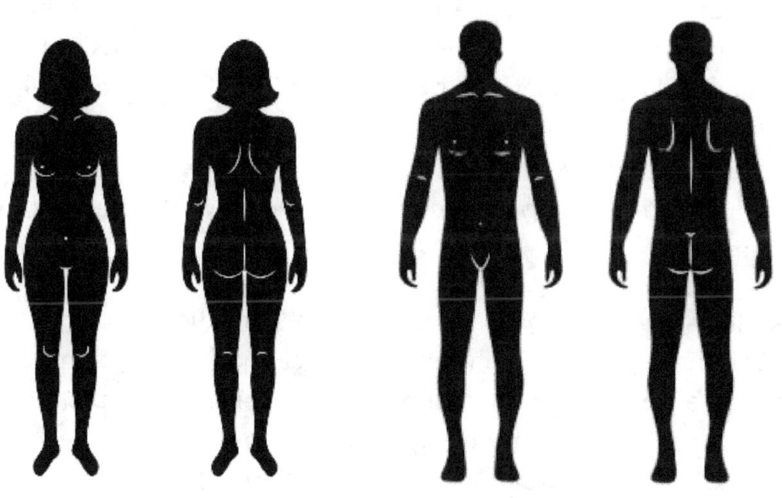

Tracking sensations in somatic therapy involves a more targeted and introspective exploration of bodily sensations compared to the initial stage of developing body awareness. While body awareness aims to establish a general understanding of the sensations present in the body, tracking sensations delves into the identification and observation of specific bodily experiences in real-time.

In tracking sensations, individuals are encouraged to pay close attention to subtle changes and nuances in their bodily experiences as they evoke past, present, and future people, events, and situations. This process involves observing sensations with curiosity and openness, without judgments or interpretations. By closely following these sensations, individuals can gain a deeper understanding of how emotions and experiences manifest in their physical bodies, including the intensity, location, and quality of the sensations.

Unlike the somatic map exercise, which focuses on the visual representation of bodily sensations, tracking sensations involves a more immediate and internalized exploration of bodily experiences. Instead of categorizing sensations with descriptors, tracking sensations requires remaining present as they arise, allowing individuals to develop a greater sense of awareness and body attunement.

Overall, while both body awareness and sensation tracking aim to deepen the connection with one's physical body, sensation tracking involves a more dynamic and present-centered exploration of bodily experiences, enabling individuals to cultivate greater awareness and self-awareness in somatic therapy.

Somatic Resources

Somatic resourcing is a technique used in somatic therapy to help individuals establish a sense of safety, stability, and support within their own bodies. It involves identifying and cultivating internal and external resources that can provide comfort, grounding, and regulation during times of discomfort or emotional activation. By accessing and activating these resources, individuals can enhance their ability to manage difficult emotions, regulate their nervous systems, and build resilience in the face of challenges.

In the book, various somatic resourcing techniques that can support healing and self-regulation will be explored. These techniques may include guided imagery, grounding exercises, mindfulness practices, and somatic awareness exercises. Through experiential exercises and guided practices, readers will learn to identify and access their unique sources of support and stability within their bodies. By developing a toolbox of somatic resources, individuals can foster greater resilience, self-awareness, and empowerment in their healing journey.

Somatic Processing

The approach of **somatic processing** recognizes that the body holds valuable information about past experiences and emotional states and provides techniques and interventions to help individuals safely access and process these sensations and memories. This may involve methods such as body-centered awareness, breathwork, movement practices, and sensorimotor processing.

In other books of this collection, we delve into the concept of somatic processing, which involves the therapeutic process of exploring and working through somatic sensations, emotions, and memories stored in the body. Somatic processing acknowledges that trauma and emotional experiences are not only stored in the mind but also in the body and aims to facilitate the release and integration of these stored experiences to promote healing and well-being. Throughout the reading, readers will learn about various somatic processing techniques and how they can be applied to facilitate the release and resolution of trauma and emotional discomfort. By engaging in somatic processing exercises and interventions, individuals can develop greater self-awareness, emotional regulation capacity, and resilience while working to heal from past experiences.

Integration and Regulation

Integration and regulation refer to the final stages of the therapeutic process. As readers progress through the material, they gain a comprehensive understanding of various techniques and interventions designed to address trauma and emotional discomfort stored in the body. The ultimate goal of this process is not only to facilitate healing but also to enable individuals to integrate these techniques into their daily lives and regulate their emotional experiences more effectively. By the end of this book, readers will have the knowledge and skills needed to continue practicing somatic processing, body-centered awareness, and other therapeutic techniques independently, thus promoting long-term healing and well-being.

Getting Started

It is a privilege to share this dynamic practice, which continually reveals insights into our true selves and allows us to make choices that foster lasting growth and well-being. Somatic therapy challenges conventional notions of aging by refining our self-awareness and understanding how our bodies respond to stress. By restoring connections between the brain, muscles, and nervous system, we achieve a profound sense of freedom at the physical, mental, and spiritual levels. This practice embodies the concept of unity, inviting us to return to our complete selves. As we engage in somatic movement flows designed to release deeply held tensions and imbalances, we embark on a journey of self-liberation. With time and practice, we cultivate greater somatic intelligence, enabling us to identify and address obstacles with increasing effectiveness. This journey grants us the freedom to make conscious choices in our lives, aligning with our deepest truths and potentials.

Join me on this path of transformation and awakening as we deepen our connection with ourselves and the world around us. We do not age day by day but become aware of our vulnerabilities to embrace and strengthen them.

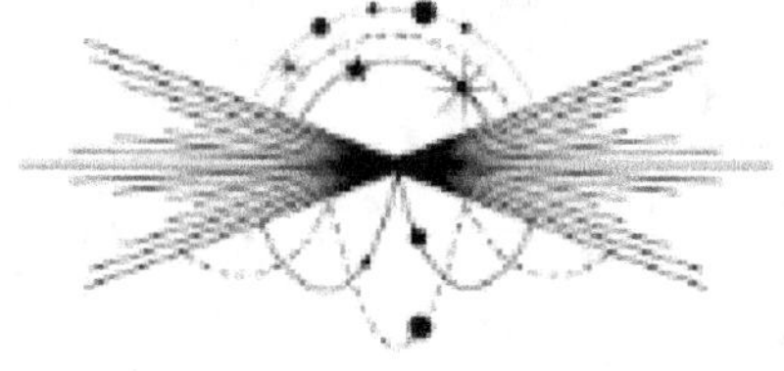

Part 2
7 Days of Practice

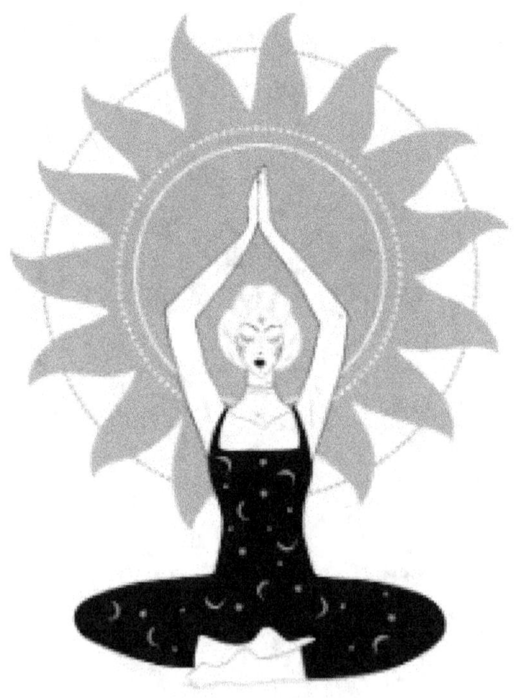

This 7-day practice is a gentle introduction to transforming how you approach and embrace physical and mental challenges, aiming to improve physical fitness and overall well-being. Through this practice, you will learn to listen to and welcome challenges with kindness and curiosity, laying the foundation for a new perspective on life.

Feel free to extend the practice beyond the initial 7 days if needed. When you are ready to deepen your journey, you can explore the other volumes in this collection.

Remember that somatic practice is not a quick fix or a challenge, but rather a profound shift in your way of being. By embracing this path, you will take a significant step towards greater serenity, body awareness, and the liberation of your full potential.

Instructions

Day 1: Begin with the Body Awareness exercise using the provided map. Proceed with Sensation Tracking. Learn and recite the power affirmation that should be repeated daily.

Day 2: Somatic practice and power affirmation.

Day 3: Somatic practice and power affirmation.

Day 4: Somatic practice and power affirmation.

Day 5: Somatic practice and power affirmation.

Day 6: Somatic practice and power affirmation.

Day 7: At a calm moment of the day, repeat the Body Awareness exercise from Day 1 using the provided map. Continue with Sensation Tracking.

In the following days, reflect on the effects the practice has had on you. Allow the work you have done to settle within you and your life. Decide whether to repeat the 7-day practice or to explore more intensive and in-depth work. Experiment with these practices to find the one that best suits your needs.

Take the time you need to walk this new path at your own pace, respecting your sensations.

Body Awareness Exercise

Choose a Quiet Place

Find a location where you won't be disturbed and where you feel comfortable.

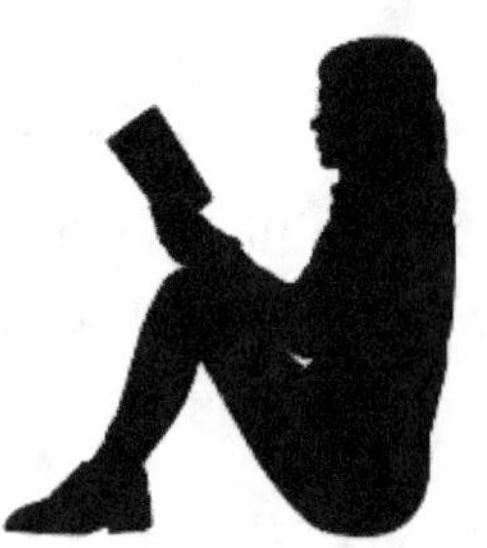

Get Comfortable

Sit or lie down in a position that allows you to relax completely.

Ensure Your Clothing is Comfortable

Check that your clothing isn't causing you discomfort. Is your belt too tight? Is the elastic of your underwear bothering you? Are you too hot or too cold? If needed, loosen or remove anything that's causing discomfort.

Turn Off Your Phone

Ensure there are no electronic distractions. Turn off or silence your phone.

Begin Observing the Body Map

Use this body map, or draw a map on a piece of paper or use a full-length photo of yourself. Imagine seeing yourself in that image.

Maps

Start using adjectives to describe the sensation you feel in specific parts of your body. Observe each part of the body on the map or photo and describe the sensation you experience using adjectives. For example: observe your neck and explain how it feels: cold, stiff, aching, or warm, tense, swollen.

Use this list of 20 possible body sensations and expand it with words that you prefer:

- Tense
- Relaxed
- Cold
- Warm
- Swollen
- Stiff
- Aching
- Light
- Heavy
- Numb

- Tingling
- Contracted
- Free
- Vibrating
- Pulsating
- Blocked
- Smooth
- Rough
- Sensitive
- Numbed

Continue in this way for all parts of the body.

Proceed Systematically

Work your way systematically from head to toe, describing the sensations in each part of your body and observing the figure.

Close Your Eyes

When you feel ready, close your eyes. This will help you focus better on your body's sensations. Repeat the exercise now.

Start Breathing Deeply

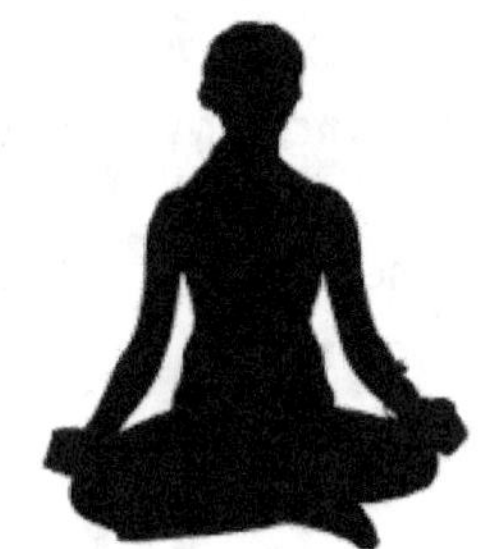

Inhale slowly through your nose, filling your lungs, and then exhale slowly through your mouth. Repeat several times. Allow the descriptions to come to your mind effortlessly.

Focus on Your Feet

Notice how your feet feel. Are they relaxed or tense? Are they warm or cold? Do you feel the contact with the floor or with your shoes?

Gradually Shift Attention Upwards

After focusing on your feet, move your attention to your ankles, calves, knees, and so on, until you reach your head. For each part of the body, notice the sensations without trying to change them.

Consciously Relax Each Part of the Body

As you bring your attention to each area, try to consciously relax it. Let go of any tension you might be feeling.

Notice Your Breathing

Once you reach your head, shift your attention to your breath. Notice the natural rhythm of your breathing without trying to alter it.

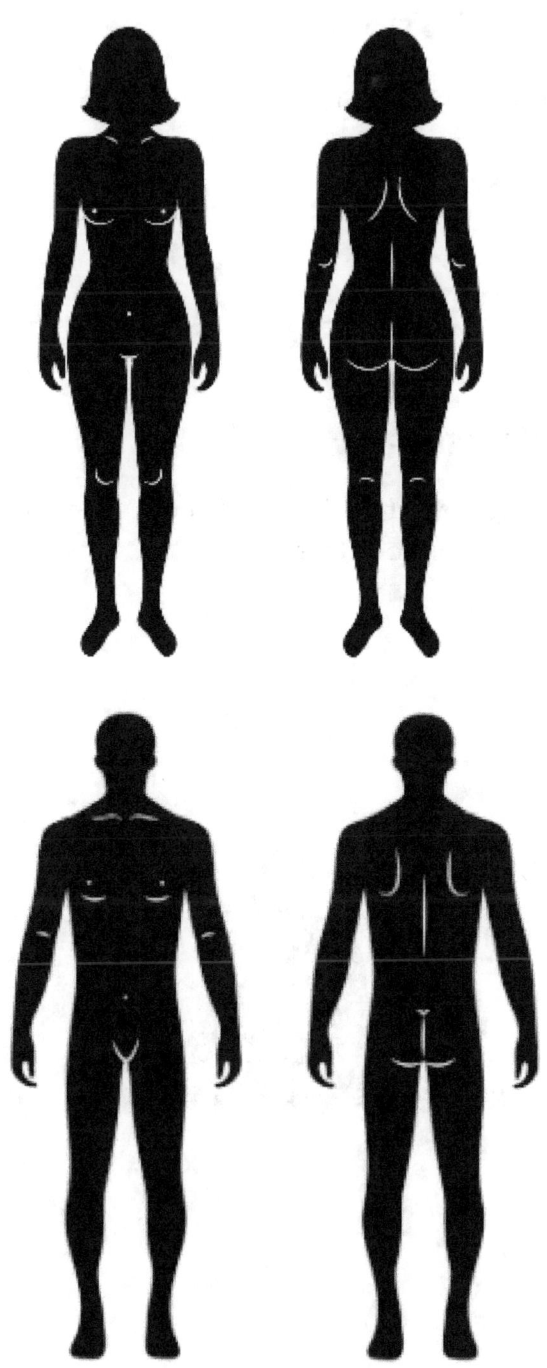

Continue to breathe consciously and maintain your focus on the sensations in your body and your breath for a few minutes.

Conclude the Exercise Slowly

When you feel ready, begin to move your fingers and toes slowly. Gradually open your eyes. Take a moment to return to awareness of your surroundings.

Get Up Slowly

If you were lying down, roll onto your side and then get up slowly to avoid dizziness.

Reflect on the Experience

Take a moment to reflect on how you feel. Notice any changes in your level of tension or body awareness.

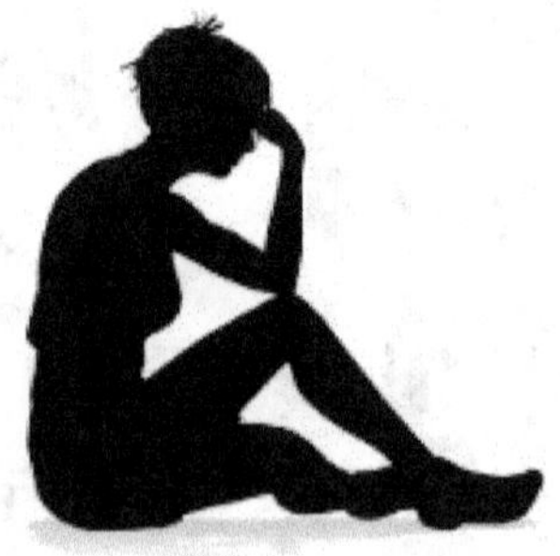

Continue with the Second Part of the Practice

Close Your Eyes and Breathe Deeply

Inhale slowly through your nose, filling your lungs, and then exhale slowly through your mouth. Repeat several times to help you relax.

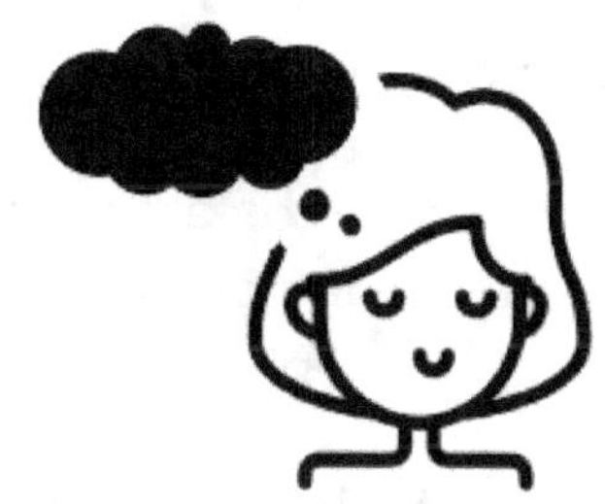

Bring to Mind a Person, Thought, or Situation from the Past

Think of a person, event, or situation that had a significant impact on your life. This can be a positive or traumatic experience.

Reflect on the Emotions This Memory Evokes

Notice what emotions arise as you think about this person, event, or situation. Try to be honest and open with yourself.

Identify and Describe the Emotions with Adjectives

Use adjectives to describe the emotions you are experiencing. Examples of emotions include: sad, happy, angry, anxious, calm, confused, etc.

Detect the Physical Sensations Associated

Shift your attention to the physical sensations in your body. Notice if there are areas of tension, changes in your breathing patterns, or specific sensations that arise.

Track the Sensations in Your Body

Focus on each part of your body where you feel a sensation. Start from your head and work your way down to your feet. Note where you feel tension, pain, warmth, cold, etc.

Describe the Physical Sensations

Use adjectives to describe the sensations you feel in each part of your body. For example: the neck is stiff, the chest is heavy, the abdomen is tight, the hands are sweaty, etc.

Observe Changes in Breathing Patterns

Notice if your breathing changes as you recall the memory. Is it faster, slower, shallow, or deep?

Continue to Breathe Deeply

Maintain deep and regular breathing to help calm your body and mind as you explore these sensations.

Stay in the Present Moment

Remember that you are safe in the present. Even if you are recalling painful memories, your goal is to observe and understand the sensations without judging or trying to change them.

Conclude the Exercise Slowly

When you feel ready, begin to move your fingers and toes slowly. Gradually open your eyes. Take a moment to return to awareness of your surroundings.

Reflect on the Experience

Take a moment to reflect on how you feel compared to before starting the exercise. Notice any changes in the level of tension or awareness of your emotions and physical sensations.

Write Down Your Observations

If you wish, take a notebook and write down your observations about the emotions and physical sensations you detected during the exercise. This can help you better understand your reactions and monitor changes over time.

Focus on the Most Sensitive Areas

Pay attention to the areas where you felt the most discomfort or tension. Remember to release these tensions in the coming days as you continue your physical practice.

Stand with your feet hip-width apart, shoulders relaxed, and spine straight.

Inhale deeply, filling your lungs with air, and exhale slowly, releasing any tension in your body.

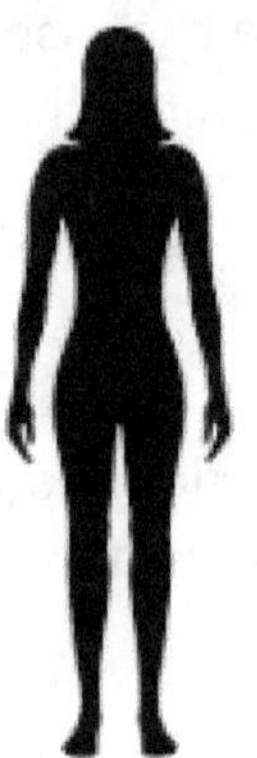

Repeat the affirmation:

"I am clear, whole, and unscathed by the challenges I have faced in my life."

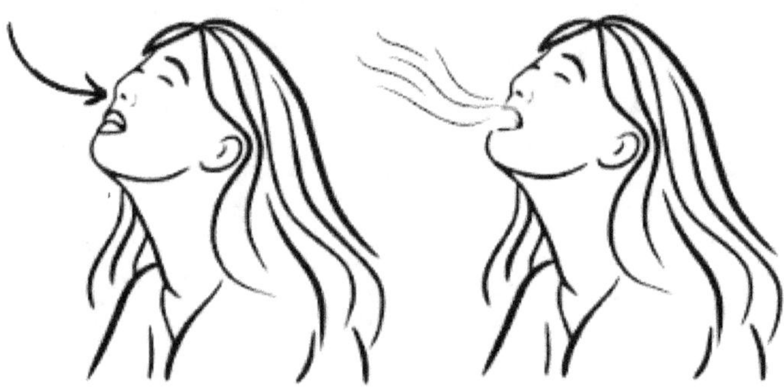

Inhale deeply again through your nose, allowing the affirmation to penetrate, and exhale any doubt or negativity through your mouth.

Repeat the next affirmation:

"I release all negativity and embrace positivity in every aspect of my life."

With each breath, visualize yourself letting go of negativity and inviting positivity into your life. Continue this pattern, repeating each affirmation in sequence, allowing the words to resonate within you.

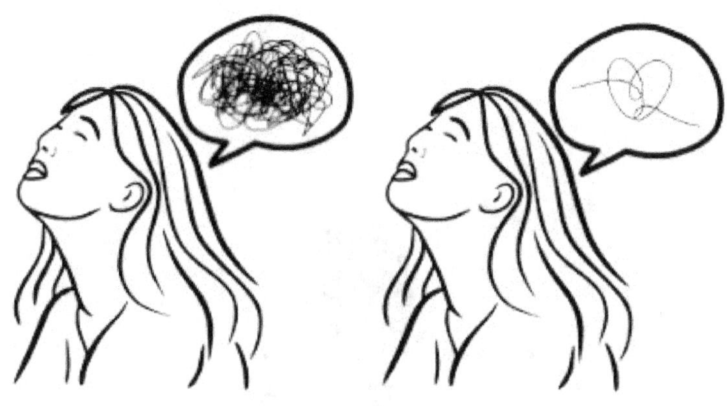

"I can become and achieve anything I set my mind to. I live to realize my full potential.

I make a profound difference in this world. I am important.

I can overcome every obstacle in my life. Life does not give me what I deserve but what I work for and fight for every day."

As you affirm these statements, feel a growing sense of strength and determination within you. Visualize yourself manifesting your dreams through persistent effort, trusting your inner wisdom to guide you.

Feel the confidence and strength increasing with each affirmation, knowing that you have the ability to achieve any goal you set.

Take a moment to appreciate the power of your affirmations and carry this positivity with you throughout the day.

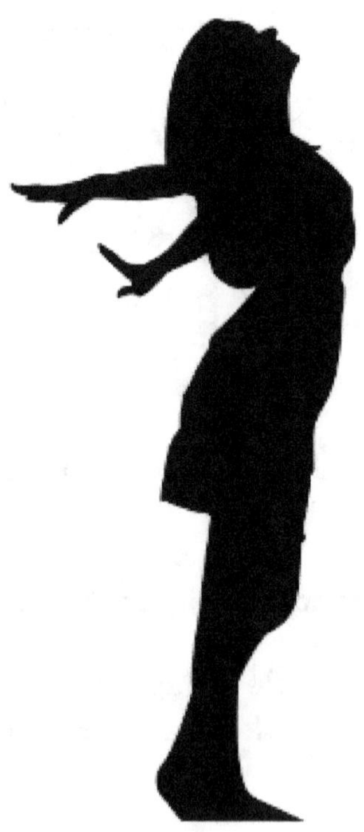

Welcome to your morning somatic practice to set intentions and energize your body. Over the next few minutes we will engage in gentle somatic movements to increase flexibility and focus while we are still in bed or have just gotten up. As we move through these exercises, I encourage you to listen to your body's signals and move at a pace that feels comfortable.

Recall the sensations you experienced through the Body Awareness and Sensation Detection exercises. Focus on the parts of the body that are most tense and compromised in order to bring in new energy.

Each movement should be tailored to the unique needs of your body, without seeking perfection. Embrace a sense of curiosity about your body and your intentions for the day ahead, and proceed with increasing awareness of all parts of you. The goal is to feel comfortable in your body, and take care of it throughout the course of the day.

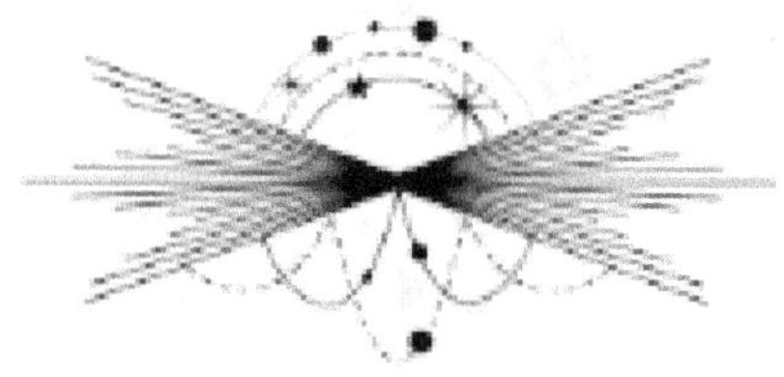

Get into a comfortable position, lying down with your arms along your sides.

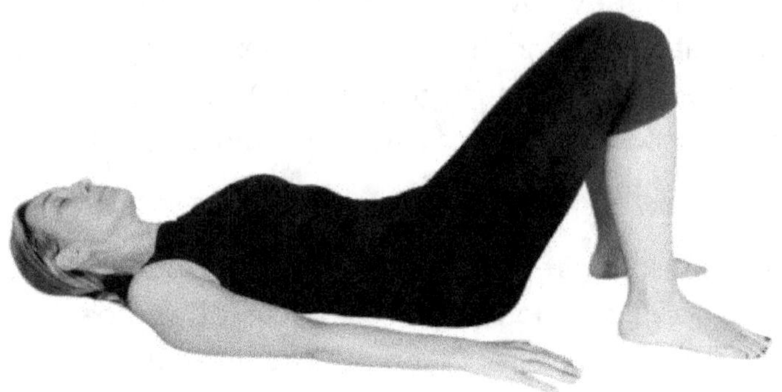

The breath

Close your eyes and take a few deep breaths to relax.

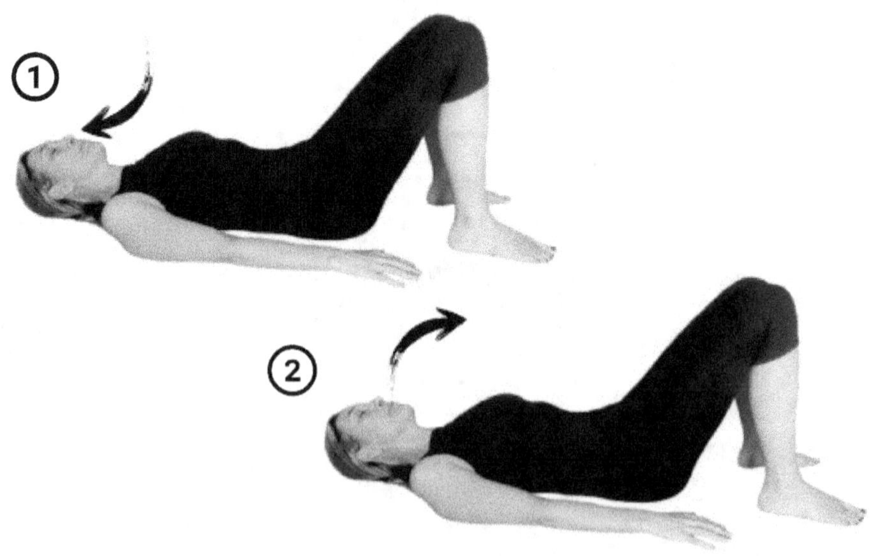

Reflect on the dream you had during the night, paying attention to the emotions it aroused in you.

Decide whether you want to retain those emotions or release them, setting your intention for the day.

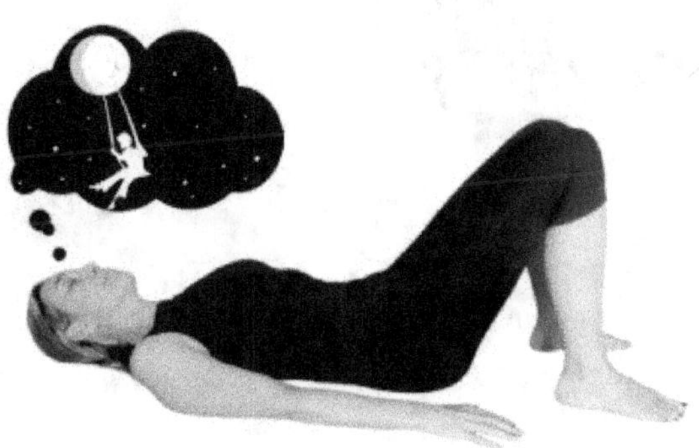

With your eyes still closed, visualize your surroundings: the room, the walls, the furniture and the space around you.

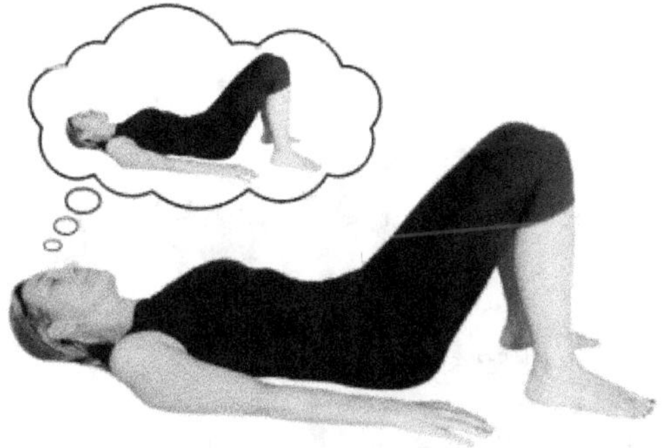

Visualize the surface you are lying on and place your attention on the points of your body that press against that surface.

Then begin to awaken your body by gently moving each part.

Move them slowly and gradually.

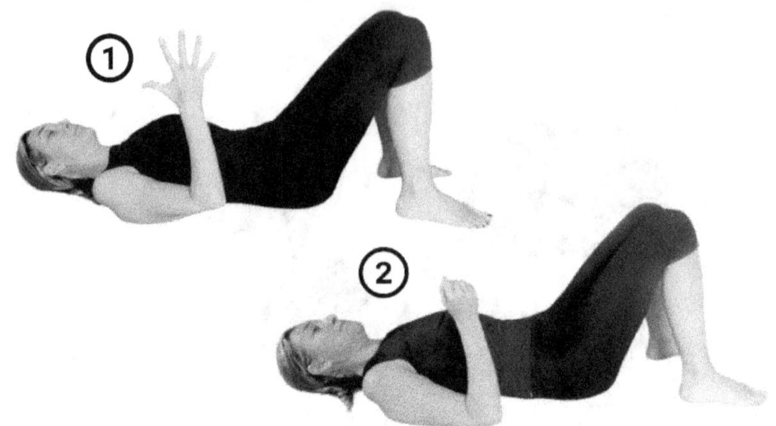

Move them slowly and gradually.

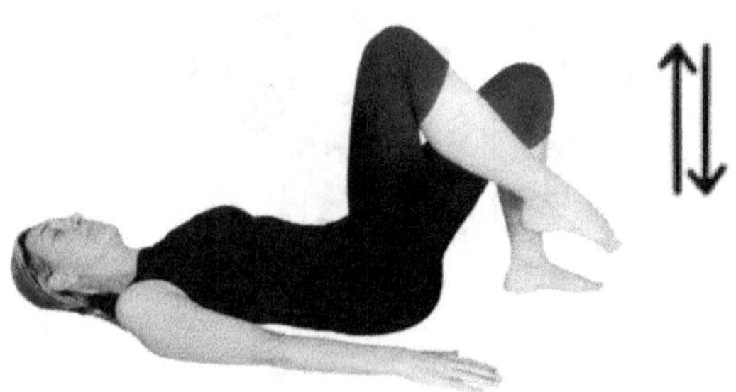

Gently rotate them in a circle.

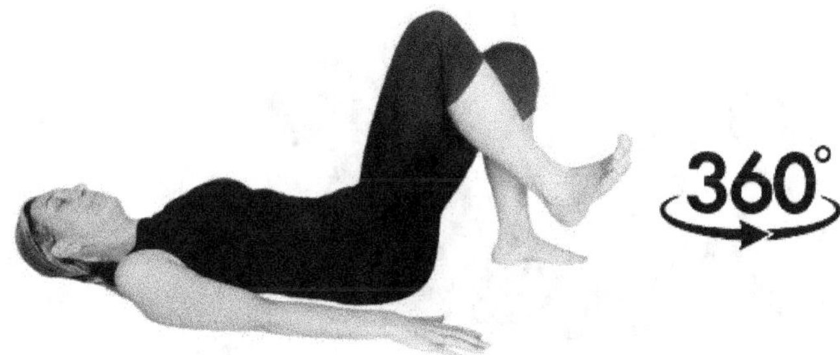

Fold them slightly and then straighten them.

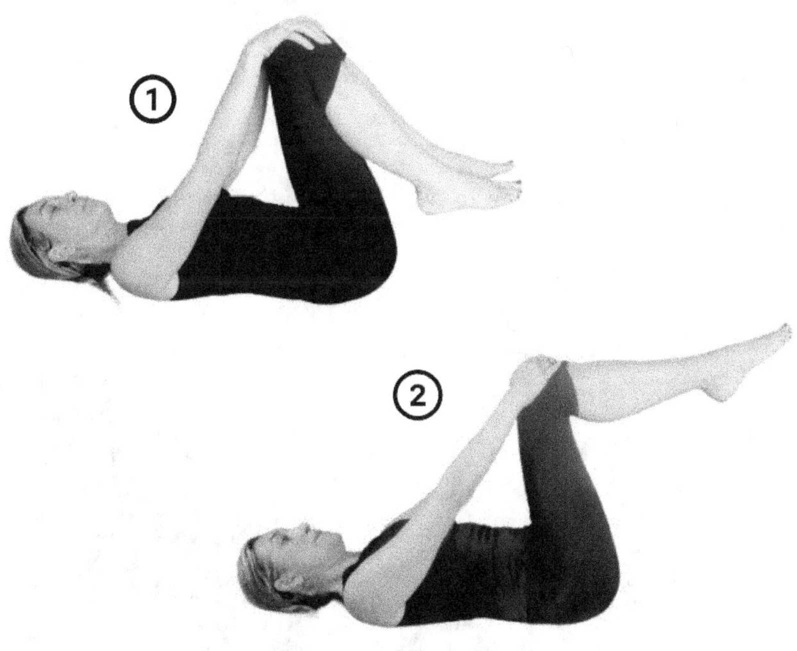

Rotate them forward and backward in a smooth motion.

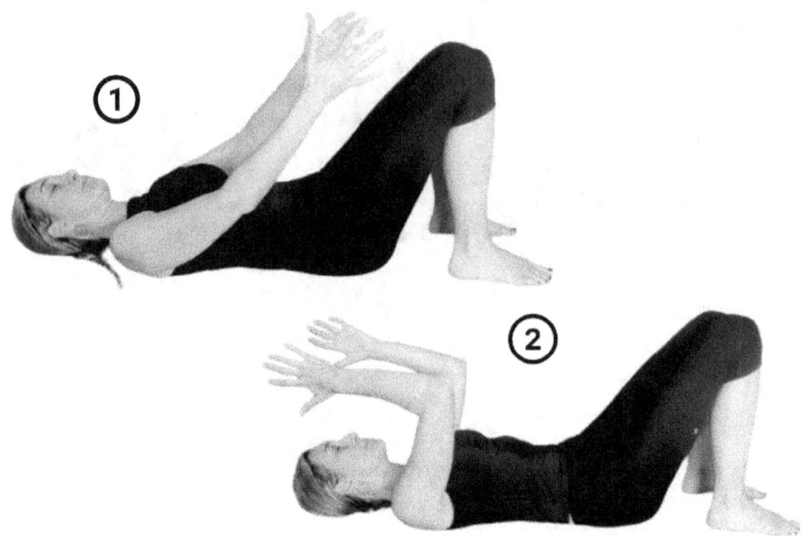

Head

Gently rotate it from side to side, feeling the tension release.

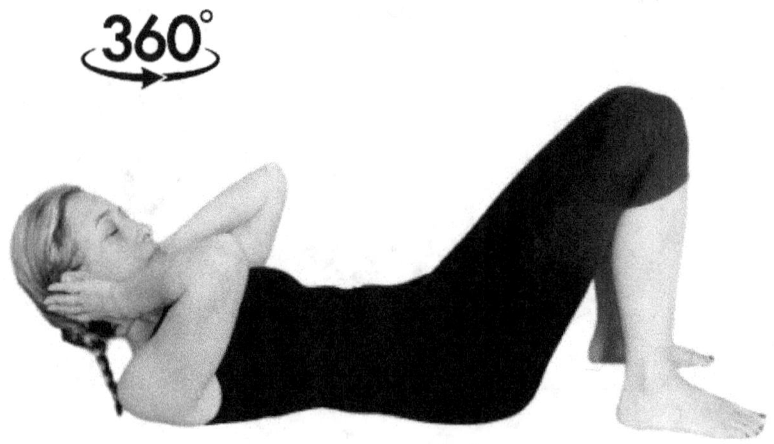

Tensions accumulate in the neck and shoulders due to the load of responsibilities you have in life. A stiff neck can be caused by prolonged exposure to too much effort and commitment. Releasing tension requires relieving the workload you carry every day. Ask for support or put off until tomorrow what is not essential to do every day.

You do not aspire to perfection but to serenity.

Continue this gentle awakening, moving through each part of the body with awareness and attention until you feel ready.

Final position

Slowly return to the sitting position with eyes closed. Take long breaths before gently opening your eyes and starting the day.

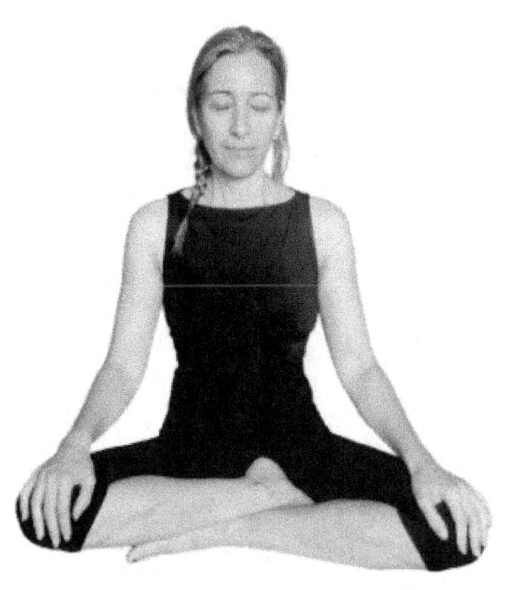

Position yourself in a lunge, with one leg flexed forward and one leg extended behind. The feet are firm to the ground. The gaze is directed upward. If your balance allows, bring your hands up, palms together. Breathe deeply and steadily.

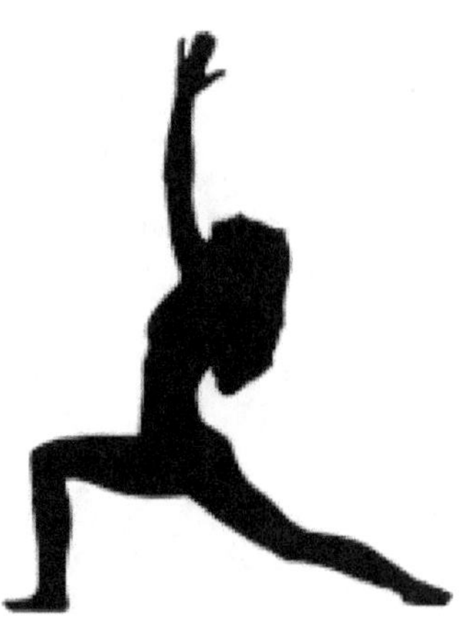

"I am lucid, whole and unharmed by the challenges I have faced in my life."

"I release all negativity and embrace positivity in every aspect of my life."

"I can become and accomplish anything I set my mind to do. I live to realize my full potential"

"I make a profound difference in this world. I matter."

I can overcome any obstacle in my life. Life does not give me what I deserve but what I work and fight for every day"

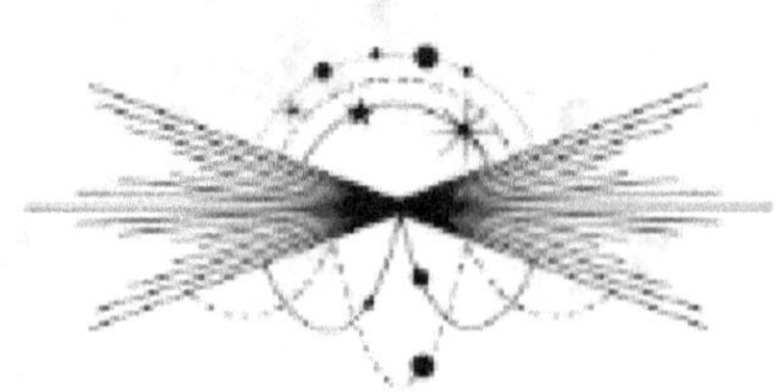

Good morning and welcome to today's awakening practice.

Before we begin, take a moment to recall the dreams you had during the night. Notice the feelings and emotions associated with these dreams and choose to hold the positive energy, letting go of the negativity. Throughout the day, keep your dreams and intentions in mind, allowing them to guide your choices.

You are getting ready to start the day, so these exercises can be done comfortably in bed. So let's begin this practice to invigorate your body and mind for the day.

Awakening the body with shaking

Lie comfortably on your back, with your arms resting at your sides and your eyes closed.

Take a few deep breaths to center yourself and relax your body.

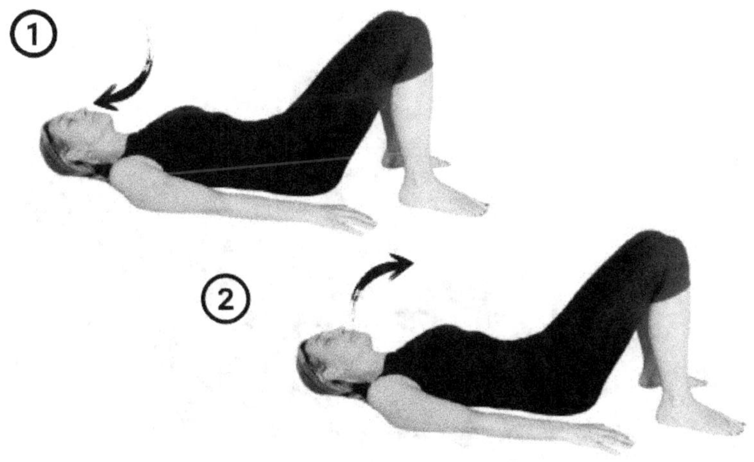

Start with the legs: lift one leg slightly off the ground and shake it gently, letting the movement be loose and fluid. Feel the muscles and joints awaken as you shake.

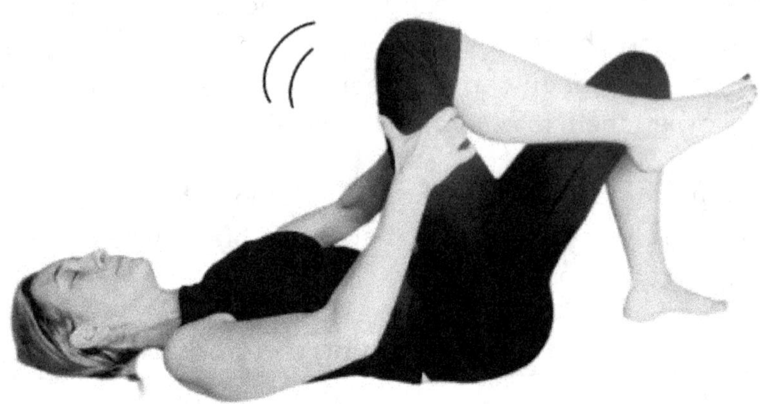

Switch to the other leg, repeating the shaking motion to awaken the muscles and increase circulation.

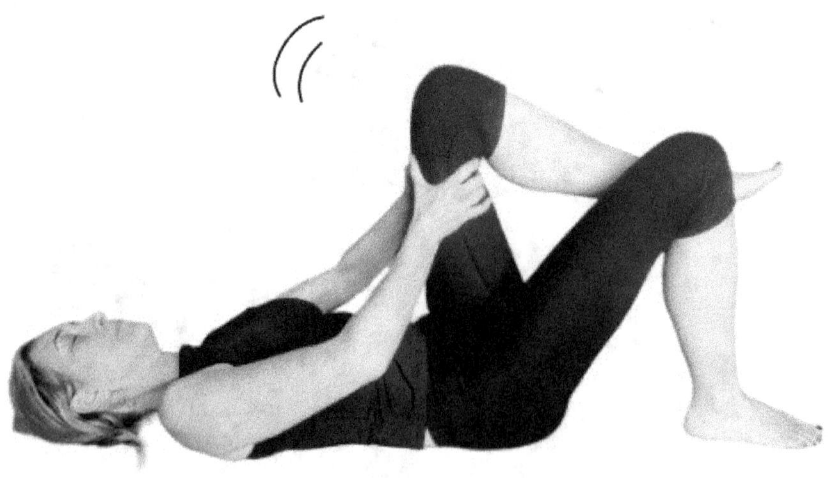

Then focus on the pelvis: gently lift the pelvis up, feeling the movement in the lower body.

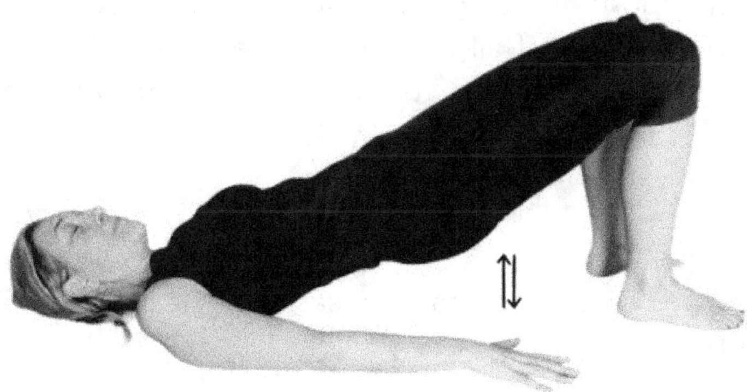

Continue by gently shaking the pelvis, (figure1) letting the abdomen relax as you shake off any tension or stagnation. Pause briefly while holding the pelvis up (figure 2) and then shake the pelvis again.

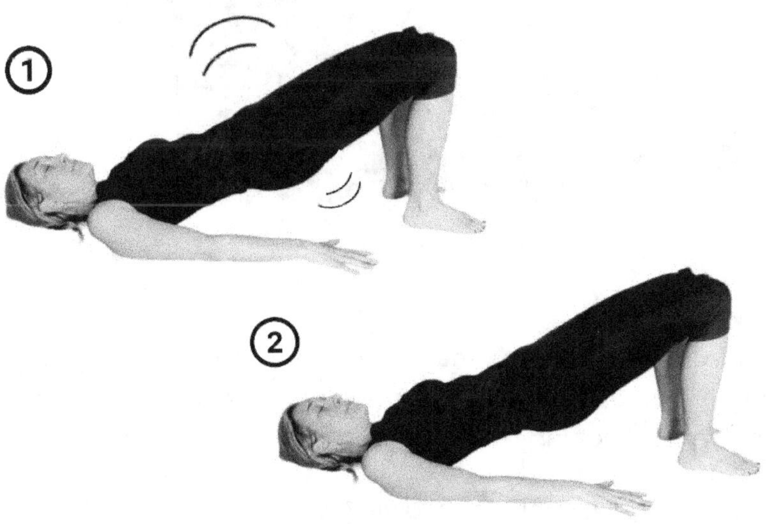

Live in the present moment.

In the back often lurks the past states of anxiety and emotional tension. The back represents the past, it represents what we have to leave behind but struggle to accept. This makes the muscles stiff. Then gently lift the torso, feeling the energy flowing through the spine and through the rib cage. Let the tensions release and flow away from you. Let go of all that the past, all that conditions our present even if it is something from yesterday or today that causes you pain.

Hands and arms

Finally, shake your arms and hands, releasing any residual tension in your upper body.

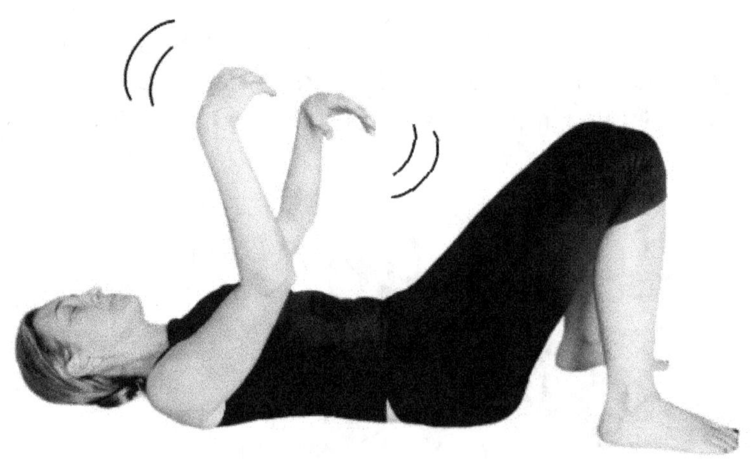

As you do the exercise, imagine that a warm, vibrant energy runs through your body, invigorating every cell and fiber. Surrender to the movement, letting go of any inhibitions or resistance.

Shake for a few minutes, allowing the heat to develop and the energy to flow freely throughout your body.

When you feel ready, gradually slow down the agitation and achieve stillness, taking a moment to notice how you feel.

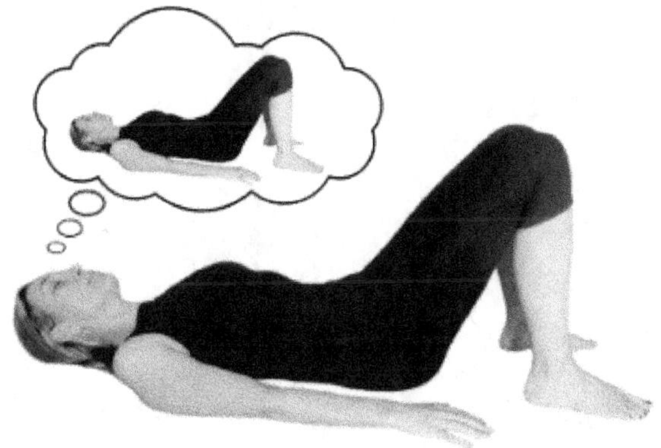

Take a few deep breaths, savoring the feeling of vitality flowing through your body.

Final Position

Slowly return to the sitting position with eyes closed. Take long breaths before gently opening your eyes and starting the day.

This exercise helps to awaken and energize the entire body, promoting circulation, relieving tension and increasing vitality and overall well-being.

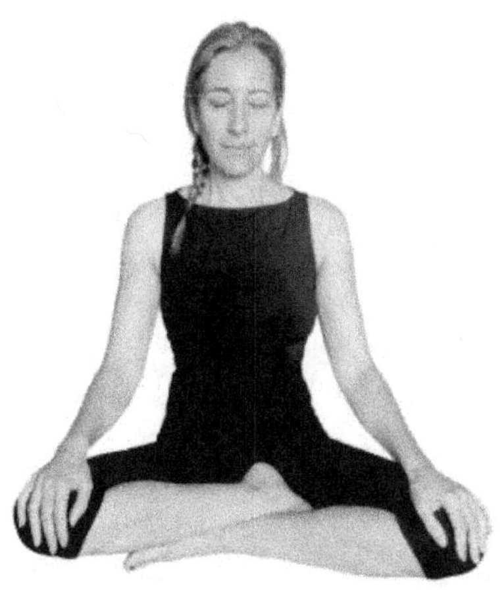

Stand with your palms together above your head and your gaze straight ahead. If your balance allows, lift one leg and place your foot against the other knee. Your foot is firmly on the ground and your breathing is slow and steady. Now repeat:

"I am clear, whole and unharmed by the challenges I have faced in my life."

"I release all negativity and embrace positivity in every aspect of my life."

"I can become and accomplish anything I set my mind to do. I live to realize my full potential"

"I make a profound difference in this world. I matter."

I can overcome any obstacle in my life. Life does not give me what I deserve but what I work and fight for every day"

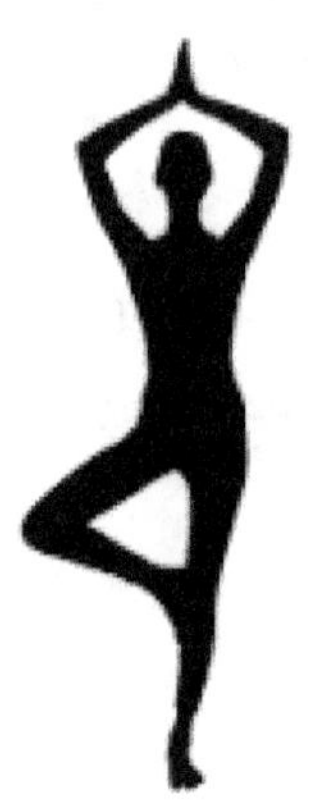

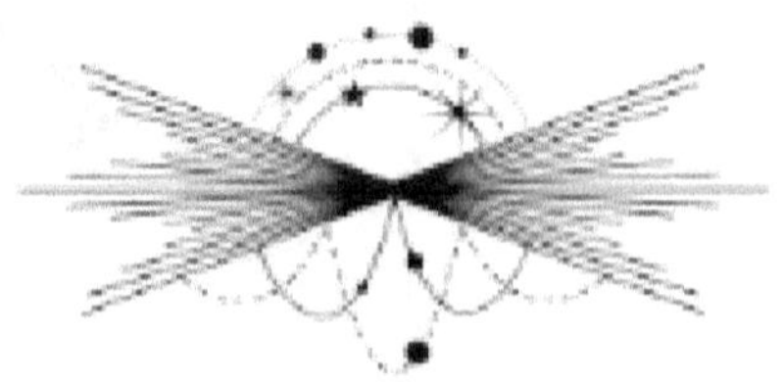

Welcome to your afternoon somatic practice to recharge your body and mind. Over the next few minutes we will engage in relaxing somatic movements to relieve stress accumulated during the day and restore inner balance.

As we perform these exercises, I invite you to pay attention to physical sensations and move calmly and mindfully, respecting your body's needs.

This is an opportunity to connect with yourself and regain serenity and centering.

Pelvic activation: energy for the day

Slowly bend your knees and bring your feet to the floor, keeping them hip-width apart. Keep your eyes closed.

Breathe deeply to relax the body and mind.

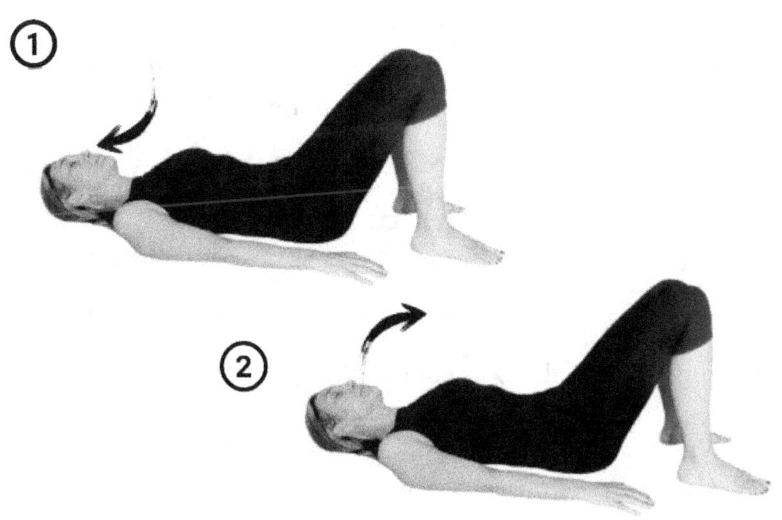

Inhaling, gently tilt the pelvis toward the ceiling, engaging the abdominal muscles. Hold this position for a few seconds, feeling the stretch in your back and hips.

Exhaling, slowly release the tilt and return the pelvis to a neutral position.

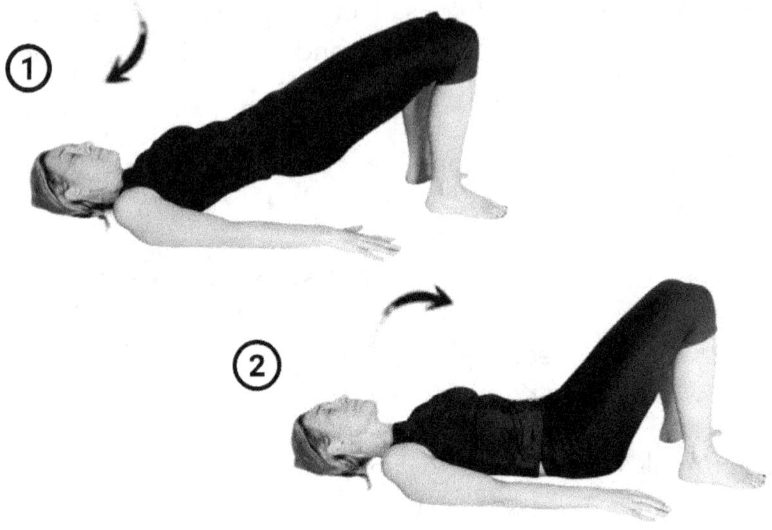

Often repressed emotions such as fear of change or uncertainty about one's path can be stored in the hips and pelvis, causing tension and pain.

Traumatic experiences and conflicts in intimate relationships, especially related to sexuality or identity, can also cause stiffness in these areas.

In addition, problems with acceptance of one's body are a source of tension and inflammation in these areas.

Coping with these pains requires mindfulness, relaxation techniques, exercise, creative expression and self-care.

Now repeat this movement for several breaths, focusing on the breath and the physical sensations in the body.

Visualize the release of tension and withheld emotions, allowing each movement to gradually release energy blocks related to the trauma. Keep an open and compassionate mindset toward yourself, welcoming every emotion that emerges without judgment.

With patience and determination, you can overcome your obstacles and find inner peace.

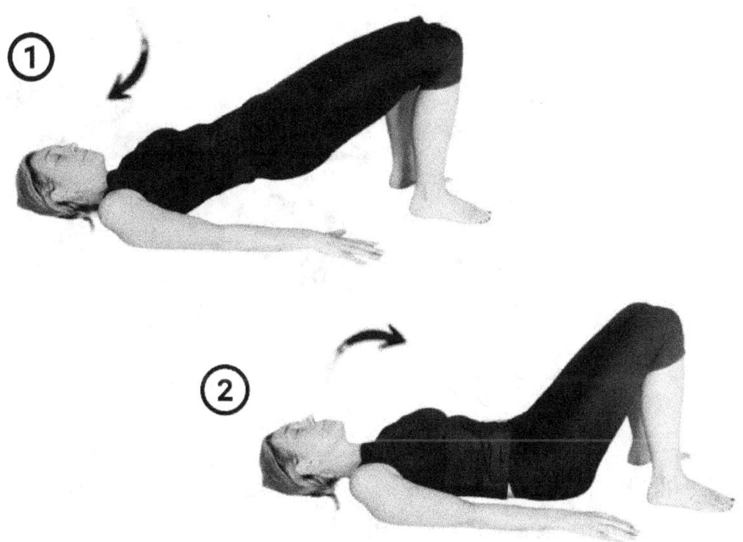

After a few repetitions, incorporate gentle circular movements with the pelvis. Gently rotate it to the right, down, left, and center again. Inhale to return to neutral position, then repeat the circular motion in the opposite direction. Gently move the pelvis to the right and left.

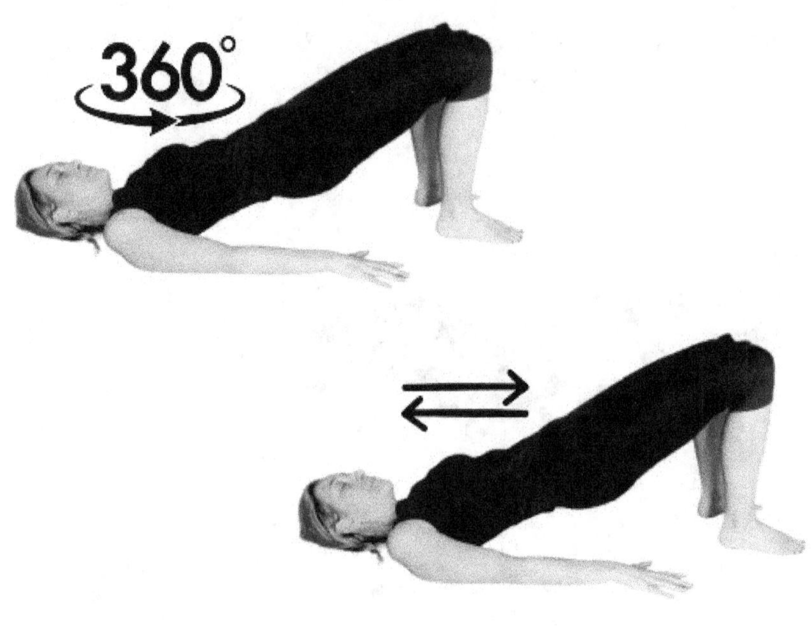

Continue this rhythmic movement, synchronizing it with the breath, for about 1-2 minutes. Focus on the fluidity and ease of the movement, allowing the pelvis to awaken and gently mobilize with new energy!

When you are ready, gently release the movement and return to a neutral position, pausing to observe any changes in sensation or energy in the pelvis.

Stand in a quadrupedal position, with hands under the shoulders and knees under the hips. The fingers of the hands are wide open. The feet are relaxed, with the back resting on the ground.

Now perform the Cat (Cat) Movement - curve of the back - (Figure 1).

Exhale fully as you round your back upward, like a cat stretching. Push your hands and knees against the floor to increase the curve of your back. Bring the chin toward the chest, trying to look at the navel. Imagine pushing the floor away with your hands, creating space between the vertebrae.

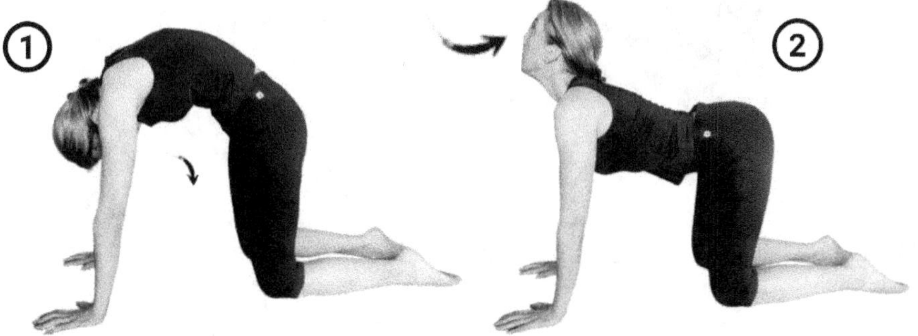

Now perform the Cow Movement - Arching the Back - (Figure 2).

Inhale deeply as you arch your back downward, lowering your abdomen toward the floor. Lift the head and tailbone toward the ceiling, creating a slight concave curve in the back. Look slightly upward or forward, without forcing the neck. Keep the shoulders away from the ears and open, creating space in the chest.

Continue alternating between Cat and Cow positions, synchronizing the movements with your breath. Repeat the cycle for 5-10 breaths or as long as desired.

Position yourself sitting on the floor, with your hands behind your back and knees slightly open. The fingers of the hands are wide open. The feet are firmly on the ground.

Climb into the half-bridge position by lifting the pelvis off the ground and taking deep breaths. The tense first looks at the navel.

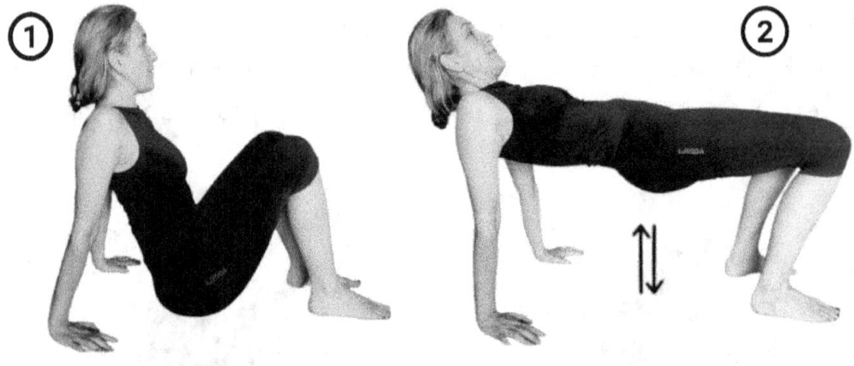

Only if you can, look upward to intensify the position.

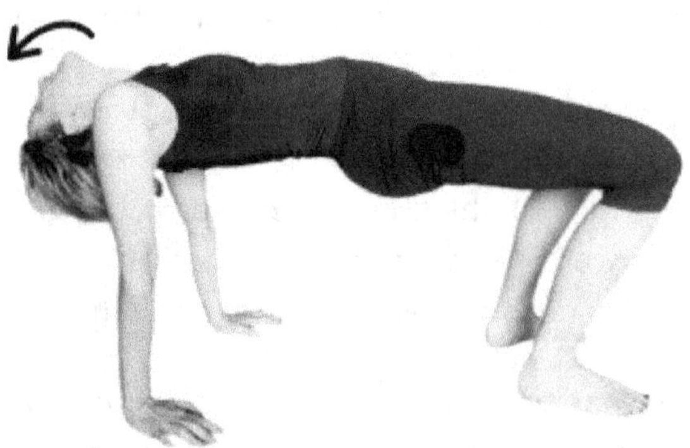

Hold the position for 5 long breaths.

The pelvis plays a vital role in our well-being and vitality. It serves as the foundation of our body, providing support and stability for various movements and activities. In addition to its physical functions, the pelvis also has considerable energetic importance, particularly in Eastern philosophies such as yoga and ayurveda.

In these traditions, the pelvis is associated with the Svadhisthana chakra, also known as the sacral chakra. This energy center is located in the lower abdomen, just below the navel, and is believed to govern emotions, creativity and sensuality. When the Svadhisthana chakra is balanced and flowing freely, it promotes feelings of pleasure, passion and vitality. However, when this energy center becomes blocked or stagnant, it can cause problems such as emotional instability, lack of creativity and physical discomfort in the pelvic region.

The exercises just performed, focusing on awakening and mobilizing the pelvis, are meant to unblock and release any blockages in the Svadhisthana chakra. By gently tilting and rotating the pelvis, we stimulate the flow of energy in this area, allowing it to circulate freely throughout the body. As a result, we can experience greater emotional balance, greater creativity and a deeper connection with our sensual and intuitive nature.

Regular practice of pelvic exercises, combined with breath awareness, can help maintain the health and vitality of the pelvis. By nurturing this energy center, we cultivate a sense of harmony and wholeness within ourselves, allowing us to live with greater joy, passion and authenticity.

Position yourself in the sitting position with your legs crossed. Your back is straight and your gaze is forward. Your shoulders are relaxed and your hands rest on your knees. Bring the thumb and index finger of each hand together to form a small circle with your fingers.

"I am lucid, whole and unharmed by the challenges I have faced in my life."

"I release all negativity and embrace positivity in every aspect of my life."

"I can become and accomplish anything I set my mind to do. I live to realize my full potential"

"I make a profound difference in this world. I matter."

I can overcome any obstacle in my life. Life does not give me what I deserve but what I work and fight for every day"

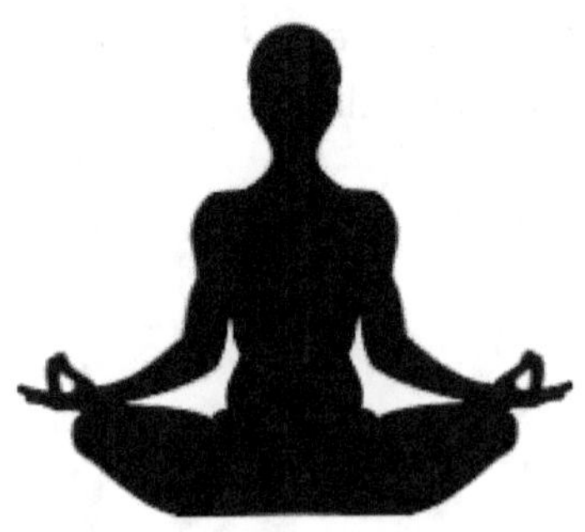

Twist Exercise to Release Stress

Place your right knee in front of you, bent at about 90 degrees, and your left knee to the side, also bent at 90 degrees. This is the pinwheel sitting position.

Make sure you are balanced and that your pelvic bones are resting on the mat.

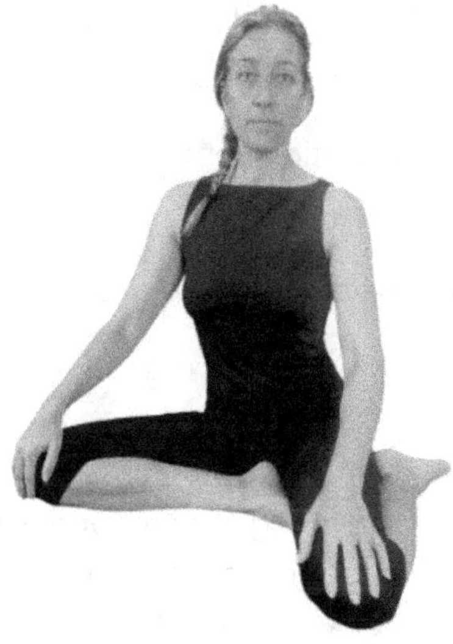

Twist to the right

Rest your right hand on the mat next to your right knee for support.

Inhale deeply through the nose, sitting up and stretching the spine.

Begin the twist:

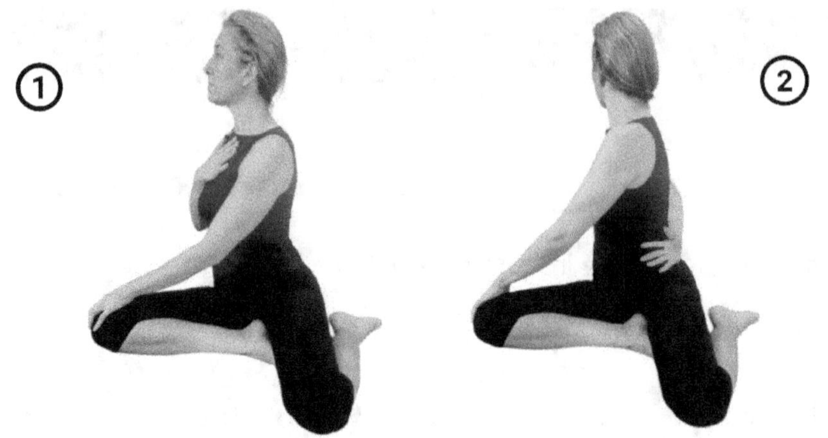

Exhaling slowly through the mouth, gently rotate the torso to the right, toward the right knee. Let the left hip gently push forward. (Figure 1)

Focus on making the exhalation longer and slower, allowing the twist to deepen naturally.

Then inhale and on the exhale bring your arm behind your back to increase the twist. (Figure 2)

Exploring the Twist

Exhale and rotate again, exploring the sensations in your body each time. Notice any areas of tension or resistance without forcing the movement. This helps to calm the nervous system and release tension.

Imagine energy flowing through your spine and trunk, loosening knots and relieving tension.

Notice the temperature changes in your body. If you feel hot spots, recognize that energy is being directed to the areas that need it.

Allow your thoughts to flow naturally. Acknowledge any emotions or memories that surface without trying to repress them.

After 3-4 cycles of twisting to the right, return to the center and change leg position to repeat the exercise on the other side.

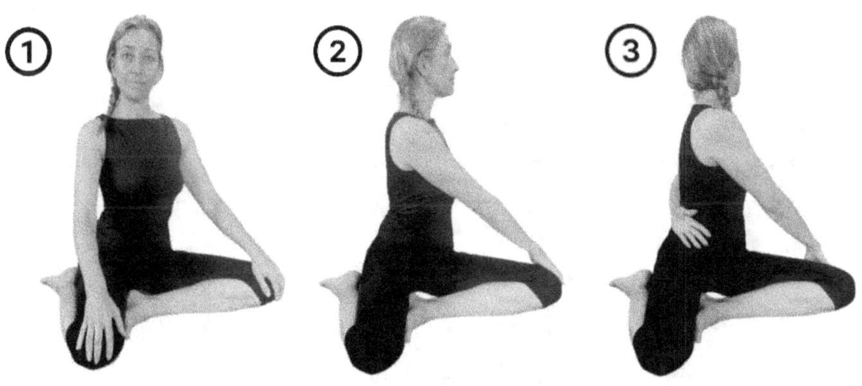

Final position

Sit comfortably with the spine erect, cross-legged . Bring your hands together in prayer in front of your chest.
Take a deep inhalation through your nose and a slow, relaxing exhalation through your mouth.

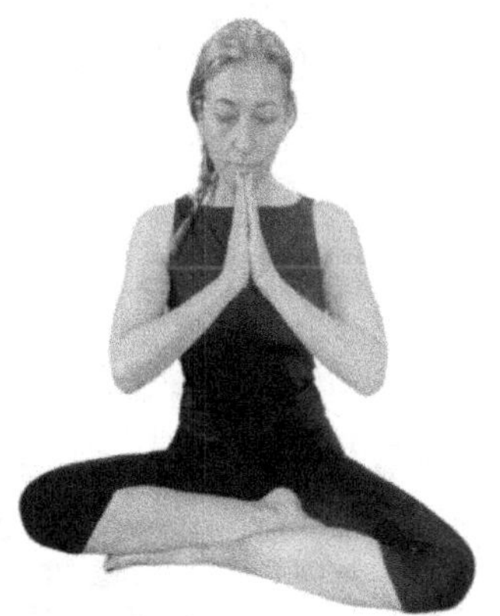

By incorporating the pinwheel exercise into your routine, you can help relieve tension, increase body awareness and begin to address and overcome trauma, promoting a deeper sense of calm and well-being.

Keep a rolled blanket or soft pillow handy for support.

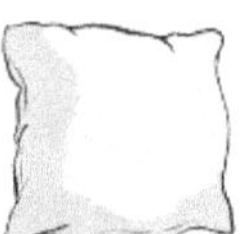

Lie down on your right side. Extend the right leg ind back and bend the left leg forward. Lay the rolled blanket against your belly. This will exert a slight pressure on the belly. (Figure 1)

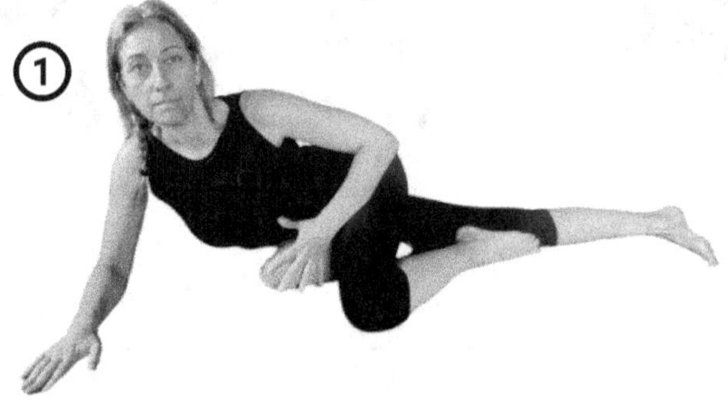

Rest your head on your hands and make sure you are comfortable and feel supported. If necessary, adjust the positioning of the pillow to avoid any discomfort. (Figure 2)

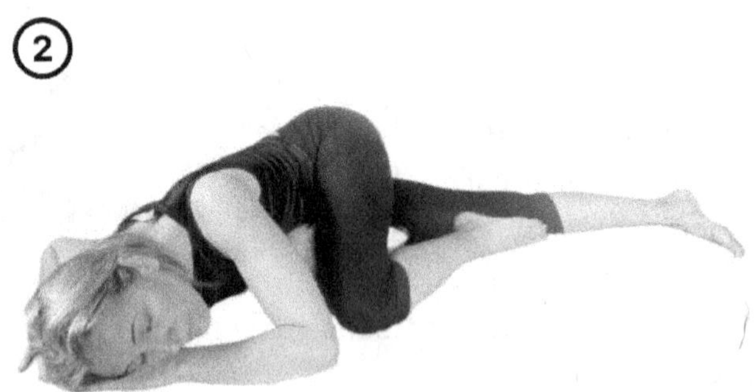

Inhale deeply through the nose, feeling the belly expand and the body relax.

Exhaling slowly through your mouth, close yourself into the fetal position. Imagine that this movement gently stretches and loosens upper body and hip tensions.

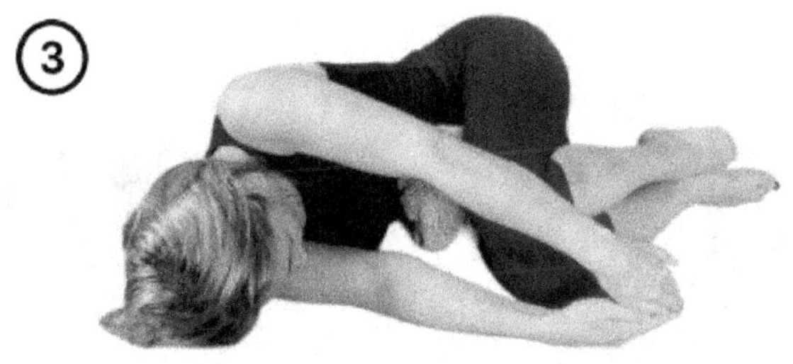

Awareness

Focus on the sensations in your body as you reach for it. Notice any areas of tension or resistance and let them soften with each exhalation.

Pay attention to your breathing. Exhalation should be longer and slower than inhalation to promote relaxation and calm the nervous system.

Imagine that tension melts away with each slow exhalation, creating space for calm and relaxation.

Continue this sequence for 3-4 repetitions, always focusing on the slow, deliberate exhalation.

After completing the repetitions on the right side, gently roll to the left side.

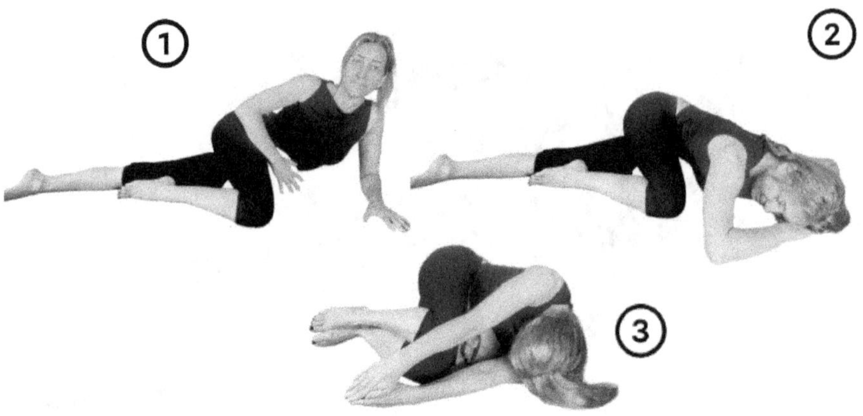

Concentratevi sulle sensazioni e sul rilascio della tensione, facendo Focus on sensations and releasing tension, making each exhalation longer and slower than the inhalation.

The lateral stretch exercise is designed to help you release tension, improve body awareness and promote relaxation, essential steps to overcome trauma and promote a sense of well-being. By incorporating this somatic practice into your routine, you can create a more relaxed and resilient body and mind.

Final Position

After completing the repetitions on the left side, roll onto your back in a comfortable resting position.

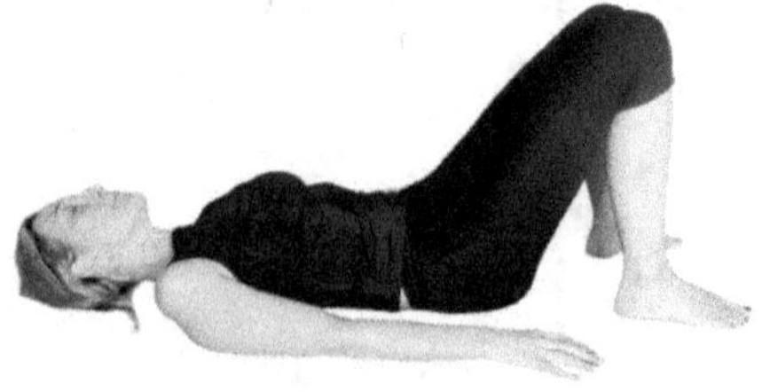

Place your hands on your belly and breathe deeply, feeling the rise and fall of your abdomen.

Your belly is like a balloon that inflates and deflates. You should feel your hands rise when you inhale and fall as you exhale.

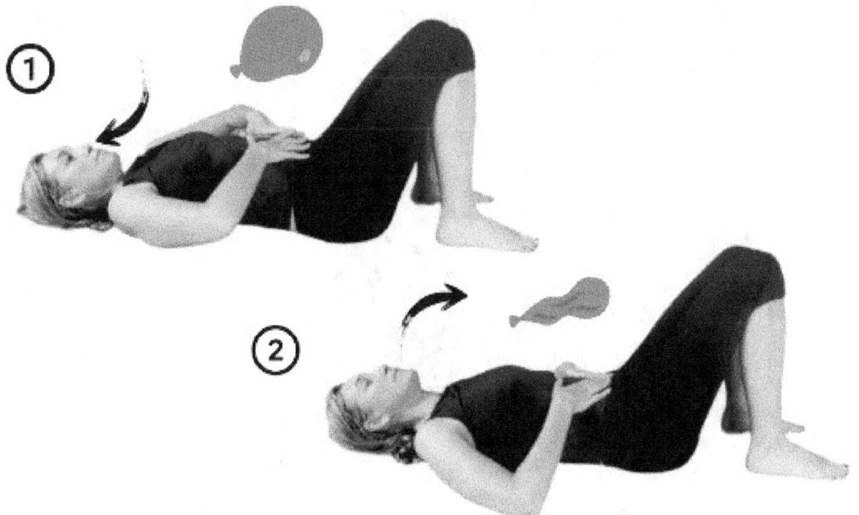

Remain in this relaxed position for a few minutes, allowing your body to fully integrate the benefits of the practice.

If thoughts or emotions arise, simply observe them without judgment and let them pass like clouds in the sky.

During the inhalation, imagine yourself connected to the earth beneath you, feeling grounded and supported. With each exhalation, release any tension or stress, allowing yourself to sink deeper into the ground.

Repeat this visualization with each breath, feeling more grounded and connected to the present.

You are not alone; know that you have the support of your community and loved ones. You don't have to face all your problems alone; feel free to let go of the burden and let it ground you.

Experience the lightening sensation of your body as you feel your roots rooted in the earth. With this new stability, gently lift your torso and sit, feeling lighter and more uplifted than ever before.

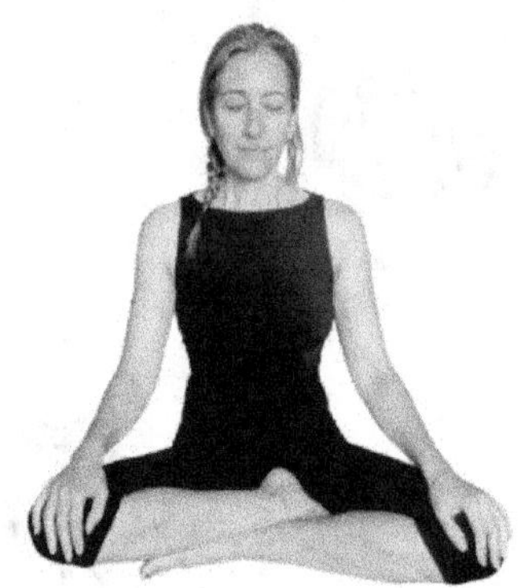

Conclusion

Incorporating these movements throughout the day can relieve tension and find new energy. Over time, they can help release tension and stress, making it easier to move from one activity to another. During practice, allow yourself to move slowly and maintain the calm that these exercises bring.

Position yourself standing with arms stretched upward. Make a slight flexion of your torso back and bring your arms back past your shoulders. Open your chest so that you can breathe fully.

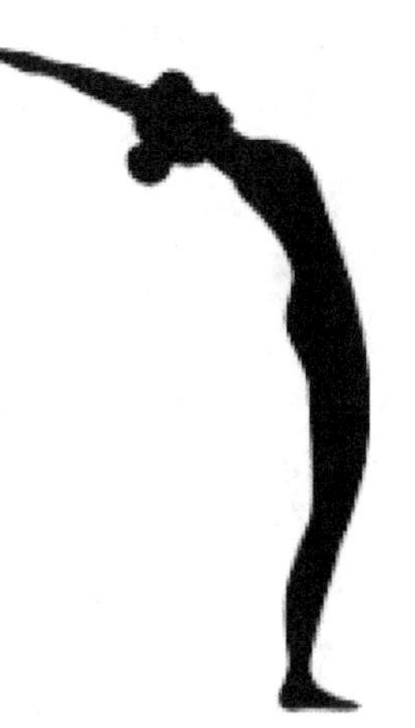

"I am lucid, whole and unharmed by the challenges I have faced in my life."

"I release all negativity and embrace positivity in every aspect of my life."

"I can become and accomplish anything I set my mind to do. I live to realize my full potential"

"I make a profound difference in this world. I matter."

I can overcome any obstacle in my life. Life does not give me what I deserve but what I work and fight for every day"

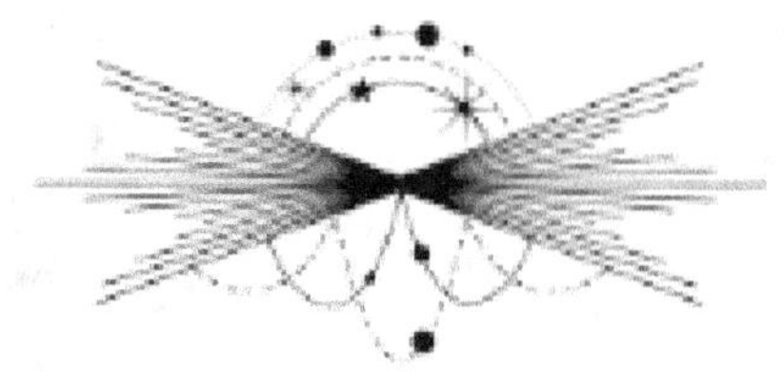

Welcome to your evening somatic practice to relax the body and prepare the mind for nighttime rest. Over the next few minutes, we will perform gentle, relaxing somatic movements to release the tensions accumulated during the day and promote deep, restorative sleep. As we move through these exercises, I invite you to focus on breathing and letting go of any thoughts or worries, allowing your body to find peace and tranquility.

Loosen the Shoulders

Sit comfortably with your spine erect, cross-legged on the floor or in a chair with your feet resting on the floor. Keep your shoulders relaxed.

Begin by bringing your hand to your opposite shoulder and resting your other hand on your elbow. Breathe gently and slowly, paying attention to the sensations in your body. (Figure 1)

Push your elbow upward with your hand, focusing on your shoulder throughout the movement. (Figure 2)

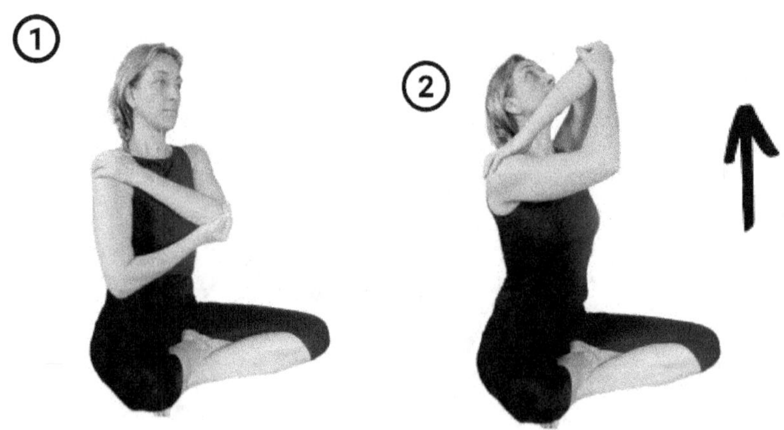

Listen to your body's signals and adjust the movement according to your comfort level.

Awareness

Pay attention to any areas of tension or discomfort, as they may indicate areas of imbalance or accumulated stress. Pain or stiffness in the back and upper body may indicate tension, emotional stress or unresolved issues.

By tuning into your body and addressing these areas with mindful movement, you can release tension and promote relaxation and well-being. Psychosomatic causes of neck pain include stress from too many responsibilities at work, with family and friends. During exercises, distinguish between the responsibilities you choose to carry and those you feel obligated to carry because of societal expectations. Let go of superfluous burdens, letting them fall away, and feel the relief and lightness in your upper body when these superfluous responsibilities fade away.

Repeat From the Opposite Side

Once you have completed the exercise with your right arm, repeat on the other side placing the same care. Often one side is different from the other, so it is important to respect your body's resistance and proceed gently.

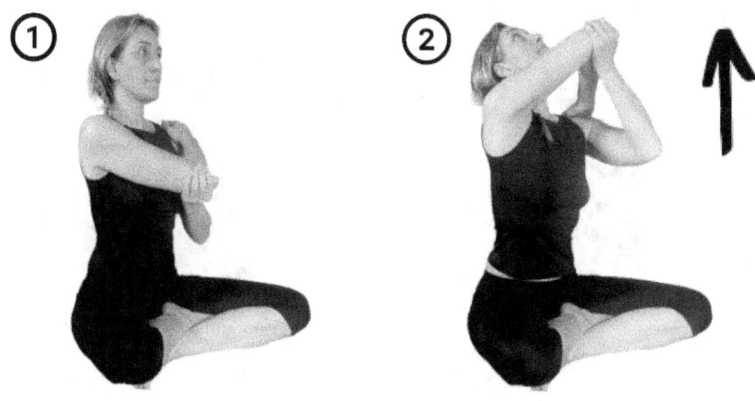

Sit comfortably with the spine erect. Keep your shoulders relaxed.

Begin by bringing your hand to the opposite shoulder and resting your other hand on your elbow. (Figure 1)

Push the elbow outward while focusing on the shoulder throughout the movement. The gaze is directed behind the shoulder. (Figure 2)

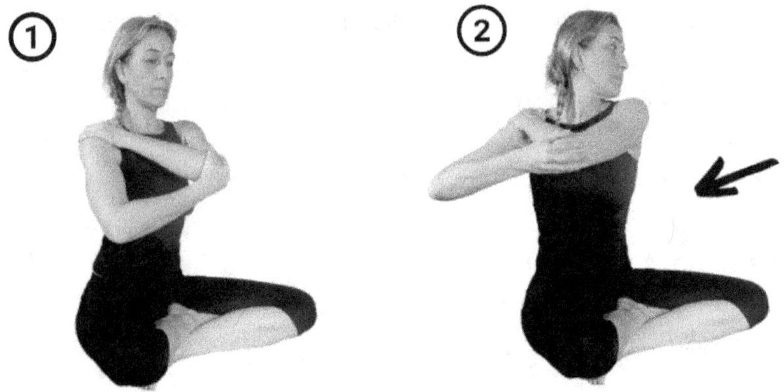

Take a few deep breaths, savoring the feeling of looseness entering your body.

Repeat From the Opposite Side

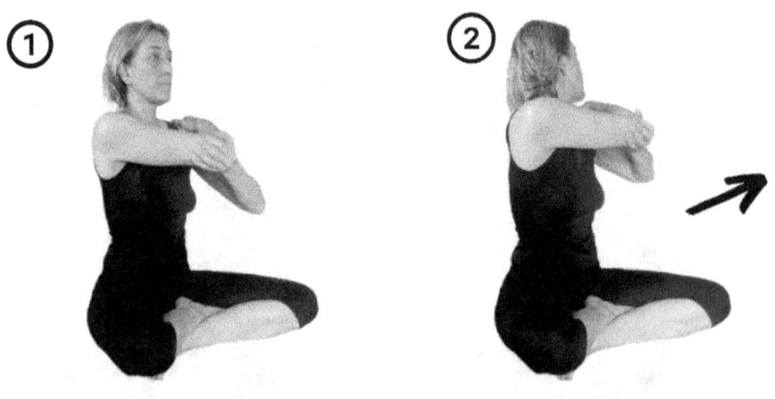

At the end of the day it is essential to loosen the muscles in the neck, where daily and past tensions accumulate. Mindfulness exercises help release these tensions, promoting relaxation and overall well-being.

Sit comfortably with your spine erect. Keep your shoulders relaxed. With one hand, gently wrap your head and press gently to the right. Hold the position for a few breaths then repeat to the left.

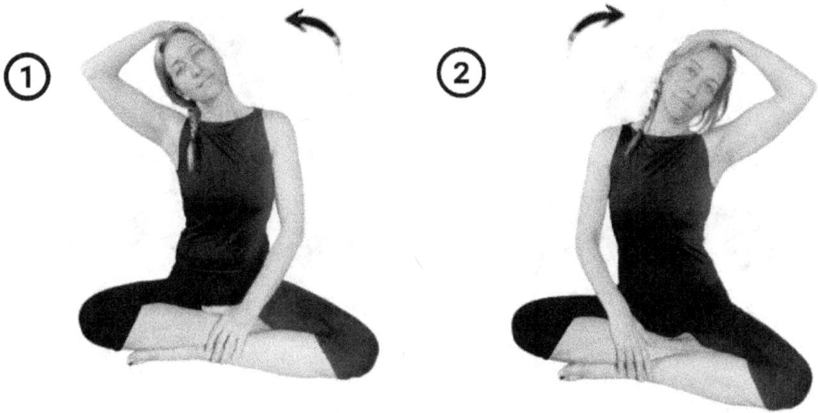

With both hands wrap the back of your head and flex your head forward (Figure 3). Then gently bring the head toward the floor by arching the back. (Figure 4) Hold this position for a few long breaths..

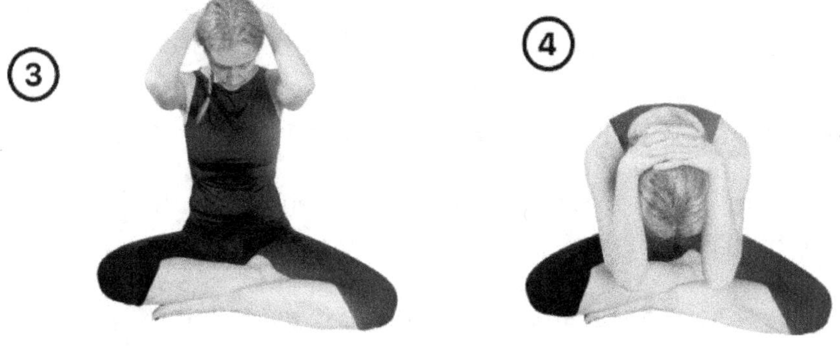

Sit comfortably with your spine erect, cross-legged on the floor. Place your arms behind your head. (Figure 1). Inhale deeply opening your chest and with the exhale close your elbows in front of you (Figure 2).

Repeat slowly following the breath.

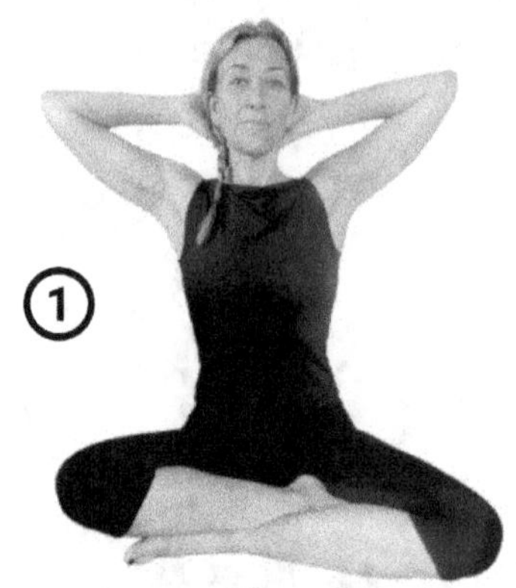 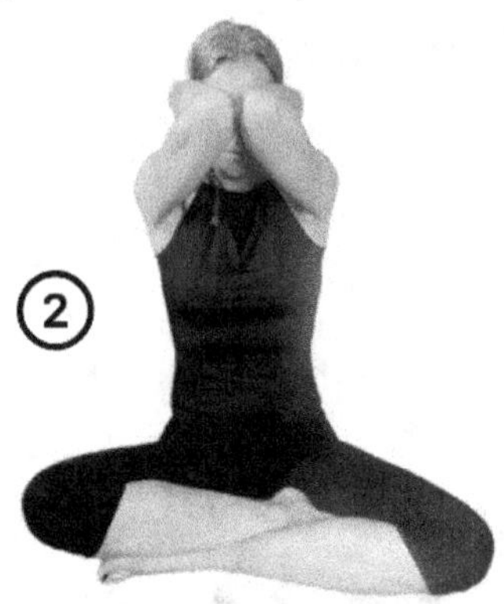

Self-love Embrace

Sit comfortably with your spine erect, cross-legged on the floor.

Begin by extending your arms, feeling the stretch from one fingertip to the other.

Inhale deeply to open the chest.

Exhale and cross your arms over your chest, hugging nicely.

Gently move the torso to feel a lengthening of the back and shoulder blades.

Open your arms again and cross one arm over the other.

Move your torso in a way that feels good, focusing on releasing tension in the upper body.

The scapula area is connected to the lungs and heart and corresponds to the fourth chakra. When this chakra is blocked, energy flows slowly, so we can become possessive, jealous and resentful, with an excessive need for attention. In this case, we fail to love ourselves and look for love elsewhere without ever finding it.

By opening up this area and embracing it, listen to the air going in and out of your body. Let go of negativity and problems related to unsatisfactory relationships. Mentally push away people who cause you pain.

With each hug, repeat to yourself that you love yourself, that you are precious and deserve tenderness and attention.

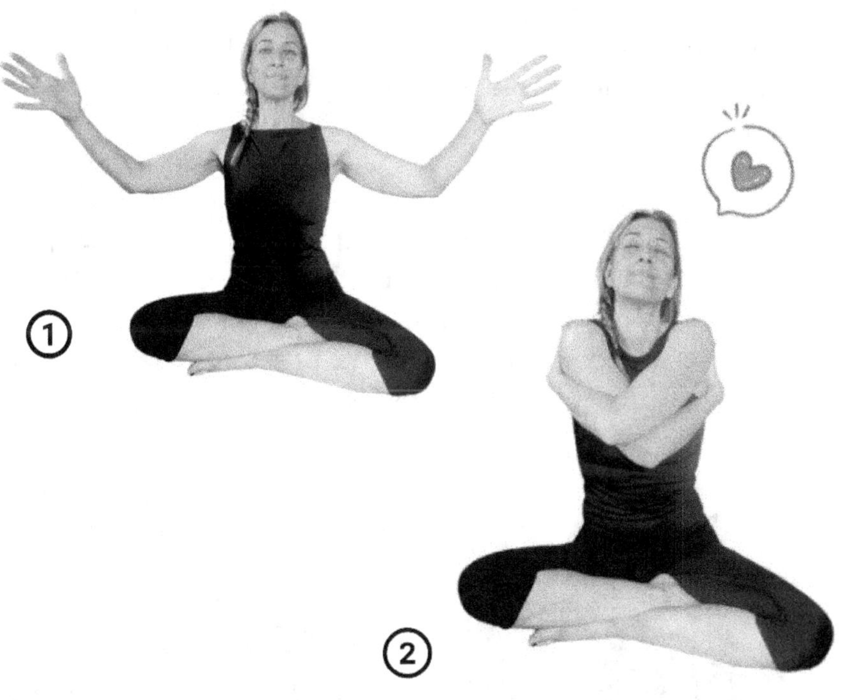

Position yourself with your back resting on the floor, keep your knees flexed and grasp them with both hands. Try to feel the surface under your back. Keep your gaze upward. Inhale deeply. (Figure 1)

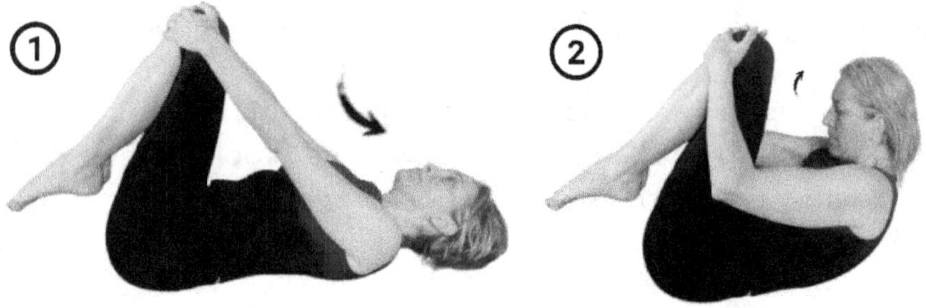

Exhale and bring your head toward your knees, activating your abdominals, until your lungs are completely empty. (Figure 2) Hold this position for a few long breaths and then gently return with your back to the floor. Repeat the exercise 4 or 5 times.

Cradle Position 1

Position yourself with your back resting on the floor, keep your knees flexed and grasp them with both hands. Take slow, deep breaths. (Figure 1). Then bring your knees toward your chest and empty your lungs completely. Hold the position for a few long breaths, letting your back stretch and loosen up. (Figure 2)

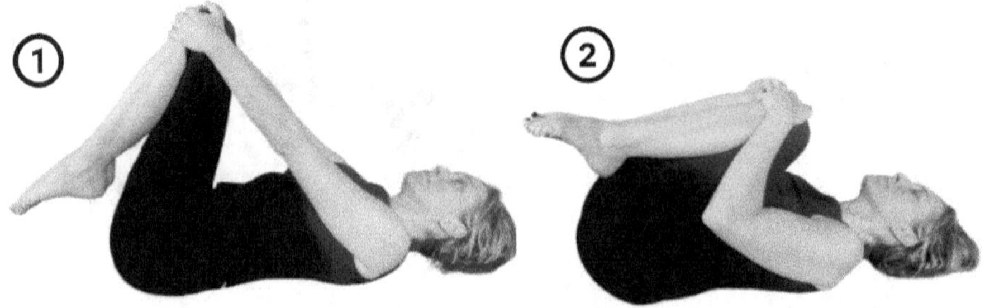

Kneel on the mat with knees slightly apart and feet together. Rest your hands in front of you. (Figure 1)

Bend your torso forward, extending your arms in front of you, and rest your forehead on the floor. Breathe deeply, allowing your body to relax completely. (Figure 2)

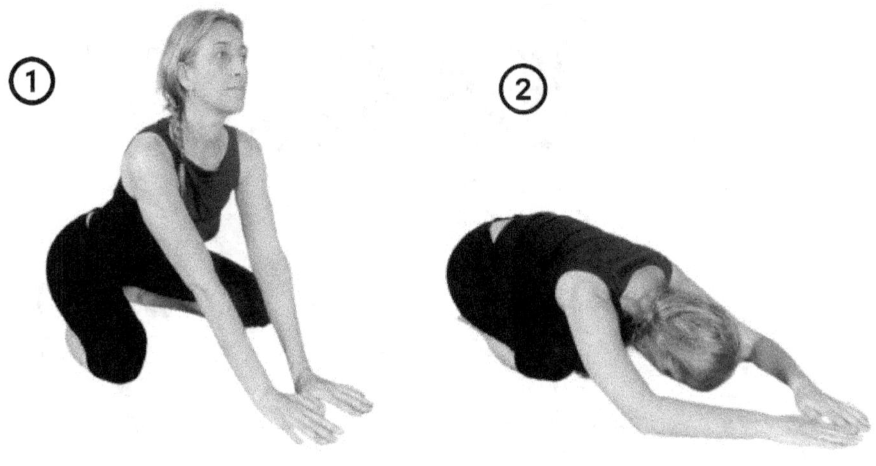

This position helps overcome trauma by releasing accumulated tension in the back and legs, areas often affected by emotional stress. The child's position promotes a deep sense of safety and security, which is essential for coping with and processing traumatic experiences. Trauma related to feelings of insecurity, vulnerability and prolonged stress can manifest as chronic tension in the back and legs. Through this posture these tensions can be relieved, helping the body find deep balance and relaxation.

Remember that while life is full of challenges, each of us has the inner strength to face and overcome them. With perseverance and awareness, you can achieve deep physical and emotional well-being.

Remain in the child's position, looking straight ahead. Take deep breaths and then repeat from memory (or read) the power statements.

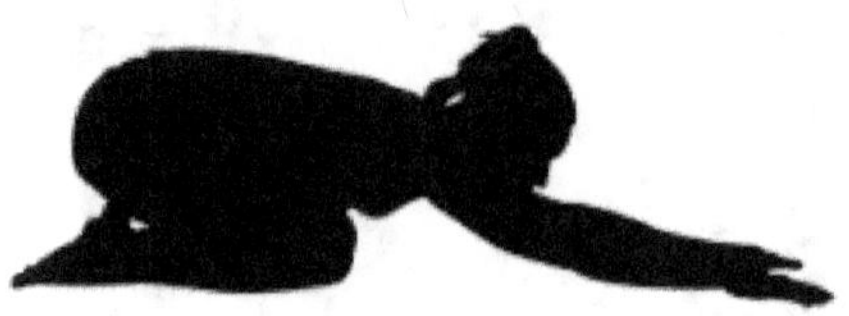

"I am lucid, whole and unharmed by the challenges I have faced in my life."

"I release all negativity and embrace positivity in every aspect of my life."

"I can become and accomplish anything I set my mind to do. I live to realize my full potential"

"I make a profound difference in this world. I matter."

I can overcome any obstacle in my life. Life does not give me what I deserve but what I work and fight for every day"

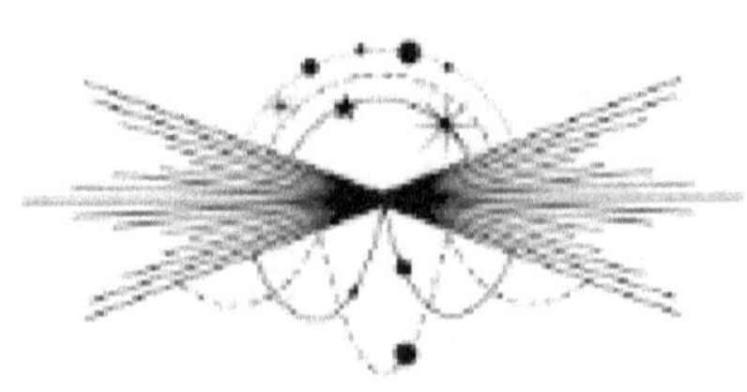

Find a Quiet Place: Choose a time of day when you can have quiet and privacy, without distractions.

Accommodation: You can sit on a chair or on the floor cross-legged. Be sure to have a relaxed but upright posture.

Prepare your Body Map: Keep your body map handy, placing it near you so that you can easily refer to it.

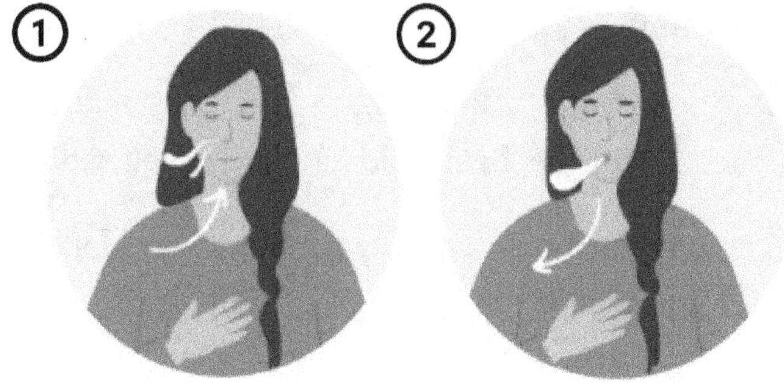

Exercise:

Begin by closing your eyes and bringing your attention to your breath.

Inhale deeply through your nose, filling your lungs completely.

Hold your breath for a couple of seconds.

Exhale slowly through your mouth, releasing all tension.

Repeat this breathing cycle 3-5 times to prepare your body and mind for the exercise.

Bringing Attention to the Body:

• With your eyes closed, begin to bring attention to your head and face.

• Notice any tensions or particular sensations.

• Slowly move attention to the neck and shoulders.

• Continue down the body, including arms, chest, abdomen, back, pelvis, legs and feet.

Sensation Detection:

• Use the body map to identify areas where you feel particular sensations, such as tension, heat, cold, tingling or relaxation.

• Assign a name to each sensation you encounter, for example, "tension in the right shoulder," "warmth in the chest," "tingling in the feet."

• Observe each sensation without judging it, simply acknowledging and accepting it.

Final Reflection:

• After completing the sensation detection, take a moment to reflect on what you have discovered.

• Think about how these sensations may be related to your emotional and mental state.

• Take note of the areas of the body that need more attention or care.

Return to Breathing:

• End the exercise with a few deep breaths.

• Slowly open your eyes and bring your attention back to your surroundings.

Additional Tips

• Daily Routine: Starting today, try to incorporate this exercise into your daily routine to maximize the benefits.

• Awareness Journal: Consider keeping a journal where you can record your daily observations and progress in sensation sensing.

By following these detailed instructions, you will deepen your awareness of your body and its sensations, facilitating the process of healing and personal growth.

Journal of Awareness

As a thank you for your dedication and trust, I have prepared a special bonus for you: the Journal of Awareness, to download and print.

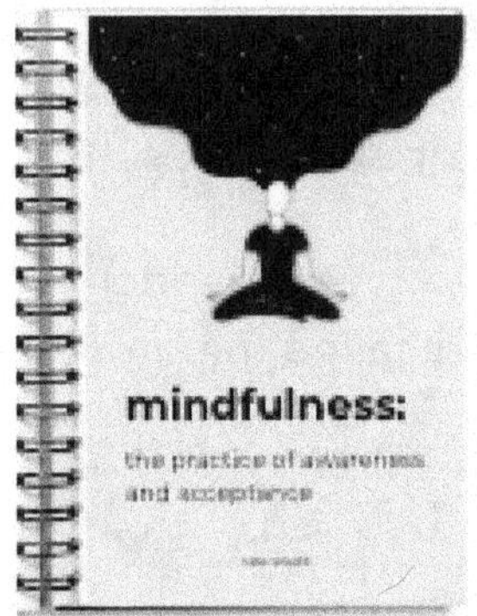
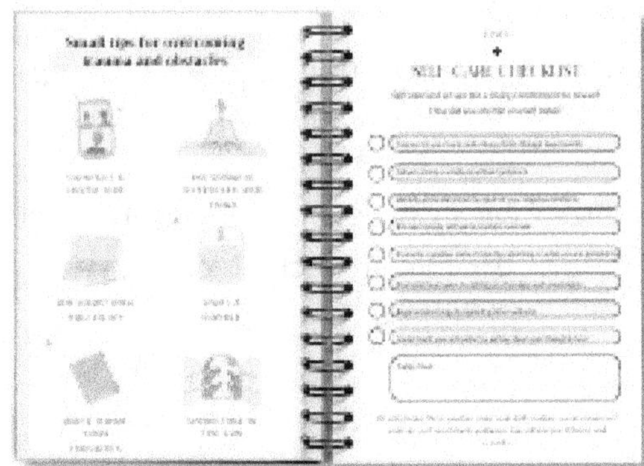

This journal will help you keep track of your progress, jot down your daily reflections, and monitor your journey of healing and personal growth.

https://ngcompany.aweb.page/p/308f992f-1edb-420b-8f73-f746b09e081b

Use the QR code to download the bonus and audio of the book

Maia Solara is an author and somatic healing practitioner dedicated to promoting holistic wellness through body awareness and integrative healing.

With a background in alternative medicine, she has explored disciplines such as Ayurveda and Traditional Chinese Medicine, understanding the importance of balance between mind, body and spirit in healing trauma.

Maia has written numerous books and articles on dealing with and overcoming trauma through somatic exercises, mindfulness and relaxation practices. Her compassionate and scientific approach has helped many people find inner peace and build more resilient and harmonious lives.

In addition to writing, Maia leads classes, sharing her knowledge and techniques to promote wellness and healing. With a deep dedication to her mission, Maia Solara continues to inspire and guide anyone who wishes to embark on a path of personal growth and transformation.

Congratulations!!!

You have taken a significant step toward healing.

Through these valuable somatic exercises and deep reflections, you have started an important journey toward your physical and emotional well-being.

Remember that the path to healing is a continuous process of personal growth, and each step you take represents a victory.

Constantly cultivate self-awareness and self-love, because your commitment will lead to a more balanced and peaceful life.

You have shown courage and dedication, and your future will be illuminated by your determination.

Keep it up, you are on the right path to complete and lasting well-being!

Maia Solara

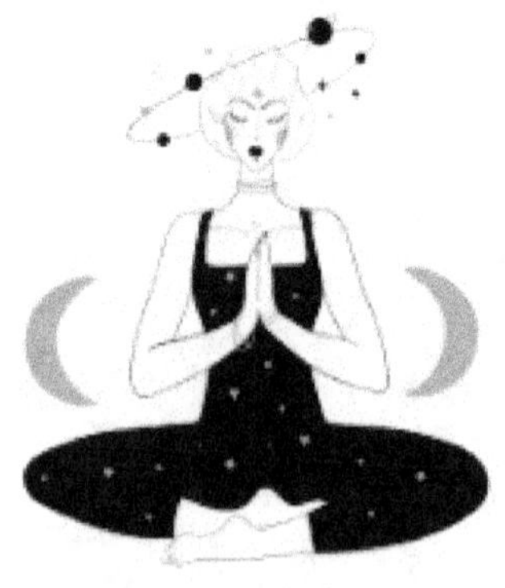

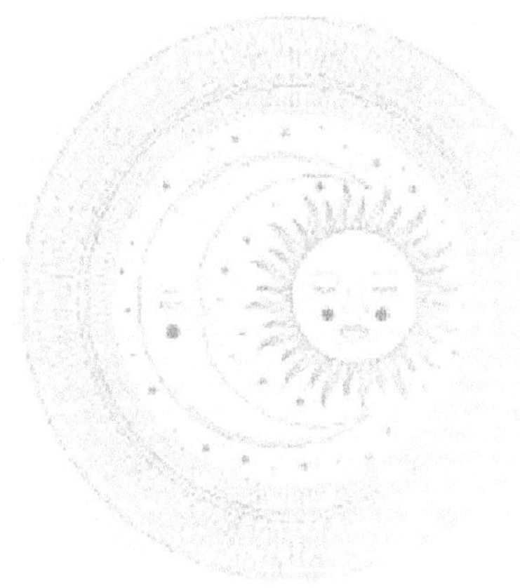